# LIVING
# YOUR PASSION

## How Love-in-Action
## Is Seeding a Whole New World

**Rose Diamond**

Fire Seeds Publishing

*When faced with radical crisis, when the old way of being in the world, of interacting with each other and with the realm of nature doesn't work anymore, when survival is threatened by seemingly insurmountable problems, an individual human - or a species - will either die or become extinct or rise above the limitations of their condition through an evolutionary leap.*

*— Eckhart Tolle, A New Earth*

*Each time we choose a new way to deal with the challenges of life, our solution contributes to the diversity of human will that ensures our survival. As one of us pioneers a new creative solution to the seemingly small challenges of our individual lives, we become a living bridge for the next person who finds himself or herself, faced with the same challenge.*

*— Greg Braden, The Isaiah Effect*

*By pursuing your allurements, you help bind the universe together. The unity of the world rests on the pursuit of passion.*

*— Brian Swimme, The Earth is a Green Dragon*

*I have come to these conclusions: this is the largest social movement in all of history, no one knows its scope, and how it functions is more mysterious than what meets the eye. What does meet the eye is compelling: tens of millions of ordinary and not-so-ordinary people willing to confront despair, power, and incalculable odds in order to restore some semblance of grace, justice, and beauty to this world.*

*The promise of this unnamed movement is to offer solutions to what appear to be insoluble dilemmas: poverty, global climate change, terrorism, ecological degradation, polarization of income, loss of culture. It is not burdened with a syndrome of trying to save the world; it is trying to remake the world.*

*— Paul Hawken, Blessed Unrest*

*Also by Rose Diamond*

*Migration to the Heartland: A Soul Journey in Aotearoa*

# Contents

# CONCLUSION

*This book is dedicated with love and gratitude*
*to all the teachers who have touched my soul, inspired me,*
*and encouraged me to risk living my passion.*

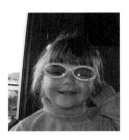

*Hope*

*If I had a WHOLE NEW WORLD SEED, it would be like Heaven.
You could lead the tigers around and the birdies would
sit on your hands.*

# FOREWORD

## Sacred Space and other places

### Bob Harvey, Mayor of Waitakere, Auckland, New Zealand's newest City for Peace

In the late 1980s, I was a member of the New Zealand Film Commission and one dingy, wet Wellington day we were asked to go to the National Film Archives to view some footage it wished to preserve and publicly exhibit. They were very old unedited nitrate films of Maori rituals in the early part of the 20th century. The subject was Maori magic and folk lore and the expedition into the Uruwera and Gisborne area was led by the well known and widely respected anthropologist Elsdon Best with Johannes Anderson, accompanied by cinematographer James McDonald.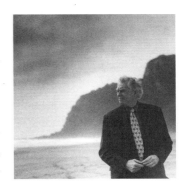

The collection of films was called the McDonald Films for the Dominion Museum. The trio was sometimes accompanied by Sir Peter Buck (Te Rangihiroa) and Sir Apirana Ngata. Quite a group which opened doors closed to päkehä for years.

I was very interested in the restoration of these priceless films, imagery of a lost New Zealand, and I remember vividly viewing them in wonder in a darkened theatre. Much of the McDonald footage was quite extraordinary. Elsdon and Johannes recorded sound on old Edison cylinders. The ancient chants and exploratory dialogue had been grooved into the waxen cylinders, these we were told had been misplaced or lost, so we watched the films in silence. James carried with him a large movie camera that was hand cranked.

11

Midway through the footage, I became galvanised by the image I was viewing. In many ways I think it changed my life and my attitude towards ancient Aotearoa. The footage was of a very old tohunga, a venerable white haired old man, whom we had seen in earlier footage depicting the making of fire and the lost art of weaving and eel trap construction. He indicates to the party he will show how a tohunga would foretell the outcome of battle. Into a bare patch of earth he places a number of long sticks upright in the ground. And two metres back he puts an equal number of short sticks lying down facing the upright ones. Crouching, he begins to gesticulate towards the sticks and speak to them. He seems to be calling the sticks into action and becomes very animated. I longed to hear what he was saying. For a few minutes nothing happens. A dog comes into view and stands watchful, the old man continues to rant, and the hand cranked camera takes in the total scene. And then it happens. The flat sticks slide at first hesitantly towards the upright sticks, picking up speed as they go. The tohunga continues to chant, his face contorted, his body urging the sticks forward. One stick clearly outpaces the others, and when it gets to one of the upright sticks, it moves up the stick unaided. The message of the tohunga and his demonstration was clear, but to me it was an extraordinary moment of the lost art of ancient Maori. Where I wondered, had this technique come from? Had it been carried with them on their great sea voyages? Did this explain some of the mysteries surrounding ancient structures, such as walls of stone found in inaccessible places where it would have been almost impossible to transport materials? I couldn't stop thinking about what this remark-able footage proved. What mysteries and secrets did it hold? I asked for a copy of the sequence, which the archive kindly granted, and while these films went on to be restored and shown publicly with acclaim, I continually reviewed, frame by frame, the sequence of the sticks and their short but amazing journey for this ancient sorcerer.

I magnified the sections and freeze framed the pictures, timed the milliseconds. The dog gave me a measure of the time frame and also anchored the image in reality. Clearly there was neither thin cotton nor wire involved and besides, the credibility of the photographer and the sound recordists was beyond question. I finally concluded this ancient ritual could hold the secret as to how the giant statues of Easter Island were moved from quarry to headland. They were never hauled, but called! The same could be said of Stonehenge and the ancient Inca and Mayan lost empires. The moving of inanimate objects of any size has always baffled science and archaeologists. This priceless footage was the only visual reference, not only to this country's mysterious past, but maybe it unravelled the ancient mysteries of lost civilisations.

Over the years I searched in vain for the cylinders that provided the dialogue for the ancient footage. I knew if I could hear the tohunga's voice, I would find the clue to the demonstration. The strength of his voice could once again be heard moving the sticks into action – it was not to be. Had the fragile cylinders been broken or simply lost? I thought of using the services of a lip reader to reconstruct the soundtrack but again I was thwarted; the tohunga's head was obscured as he commanded the sticks to move forward.

To me, this was a true record of Aotearoa's mysterious and amazing spiritual past. Years later, when I was finishing my book on the Waitakere coastline, I took time to read records of the Maori past and gradually I started to uncover another layer of a spiritual mystic presence that imbued this part of my world: the ancient pa sites, the sacred groves where bodies (following death) would lay waiting for the bones to be scraped before being taken to the high cliffs above the coastline, coated in red ochre and clay in carved boxes, to be kept in tapu space. Here again was a world that held so much mystery.

Michael Parmenter, the extraordinary New Zealand dancer, relates that while learning and training in the ancient art of Butoh Dance in Japan, he was taken from the dojo up into the mountains behind the village and, as part of his training and immersion, given a small vessel of water and instructed to climb to a high cave, where he would lay for a week with only the water for sustenance. The purpose was to reach into his inner most self and, as the days and nights rolled together, he would become part of both the past and the future. I felt in some ways this might be the link I too was looking for: an ancient spiritual journey within the self to understand the hidden world of spiritual understanding and touch the planes of our existence.

And so I did exactly that, I returned to a high cave screened by a vast pohutukawa tree in the cliffs between Karekare and the Pararaha Valley. Here I entered a new existence I never knew could be accessed: one of concentration, of despair, of life and death. And to me came a new sense of contact beyond a veiled world. I consider this an experience one can have in New Zealand; for this land is new and yet it is old. The land is crossed by many lines, walking tracks that have seen journeys towards war and acquisition – of ownership and mana. These are our lay lines. In Europe these ancient lay lines, beaten by thousands of feet, were the sites of pagan rituals. They were used by Roman and conquering armies following the exact same routes. In later times, cathedrals were built on these sites. They were always given sacred significance; magical insight was thought to have taken place along their sides and intersections. In New Zealand, where one of these lay lines crosses into the ocean, it is believed psychic phenomena appear as almost everyday occurrences. I heard an interesting radio programme about five conservation workers restoring the old 19th century lighthouse at Potu, guarding the entrance to the Kaipara Heads. They were painting and renewing the lighthouse timbers on a windy blustery west coast day when they observed, far down below, the arrival of a rowboat with five or six people on board. They also noticed there was no larger vessel visible, from which the rowboat could have come, and it occurred to them the harbour was rather rough for a boat to be out. They watched the boat coming ashore below the lighthouse and expected those on board to come up the four to five hundred metres to inspect their work. Nobody arrived, and when they looked again for the boat it was nowhere to be seen. Indeed, it never existed.

I was so fascinated by this story I went and camped at the lighthouse. For two days I enjoyed the glorious view, the serenity, the roaring wind and the sense of wonder. And then it happened. On the third morning, while cooking breakfast I glimpsed through the trees a group of people moving quietly in coloured clothes, filtered by the sunlight and I clearly heard the twittering of voices. I thought I could clearly distinguish children's voices. I was taken by surprise and expected a family group to come through the trees and share a story or a cup of tea. I stood awaiting them but they simply never appeared. My friend and companion on this trip was sitting in the sun below the lighthouse and later joined me. I asked him if he had seen a group of trampers or a family coming up to the lighthouse from the sand dunes. He looked at me bewildered and assured me no one had come up the dunes or had been walking the beach in the last hour.

How do these stories connect? What is this country capable of delivering? What mysteries does it hold? I am certainly someone who has never seen a flying saucer or even a ghost, I'm just not in that realm of expectation, but I do have a deep sense of place and what possibilities can be. The land to me holds its secrets close and I think there are ways one can access an elusive chapter of the past. Even in a world of pace and pressure there is another reality that is a parallel universe, close to the one in which we exist. The mind has to be kept open and accepting. There is a place and a time to move closer to our own existence, to understand that even as we watch a sunset, waiting for the phenomenon of the green flash on the west horizon, that fleeting instant can hold eons of secrets. I have spent my life expecting the unexpected and it's disappointing this attitude seems to have drifted away from our psyche. I have chosen to spend much of my life at one place – Karekare, on Auckland's west coast. I know each rock and I understand its long and rich history, its bloody past. And in a way, I have become part of that place and been able to resolve and heal some of the grief that has surrounded its Maori tragedy. While treating with huge respect and aroha that historic chapter in this place, I also feel it gives a sense of what exists now and what has existed in the past. It's an essence really that comes, not only at an unexpected moment, but which can touch our very being while surfing, swimming or walking, or just sitting on the beach. These are special and significant moments in our lives.

I will never, I don't think, be able to unravel the mystery of the tohunga and his craft for telling the outcome of battle, but I can appreciate its truth: once people walked on this Earth and this land that had at their fingertips, deep and ancient mysteries.

New Zealand has an underlying consciousness which makes us able and capable of tapping into this mystery and history, to carry it into the future and pass it on to future generations. Much of my life has been a journey of discovering the ability of ordinary people to do extraordinary things, and although I think anyone on this planet is capable of this, somehow New Zealand has the energy, a magnetic field that's new and fresh and easier to access. That to me is good enough to give it the acknowledgement and the dignity as unique in the world. We can be teachers of wisdom, of mystery and of soul politics, of environmental truth and consciousness. We can wear the cloak of mana and carry the mantle of wise and good facilitators. I believe we are the inheritors of more than dreams and visions. We are able to resonate the past into the future, and that is the connection I want to pass on to future generations.

# INTRODUCTION

## How Love-in-action is seeding a Whole New World

This book is an inquiry into the questions:

*What does it mean to live your passion?*
*How does living your passion become Love-in-action?*
*How does Love-in-action seed a whole new world?*

I have been living these questions in various ways for twenty-five years, and they led me to New Zealand in 1994. In March 2007, I began to ask these questions in what became a series of nineteen interviews with twenty four people, all of whom are involved in their own unique ways, in creating a new way forward for humanity.

I have chosen to focus on New Zealand, not only because it has been my home for the last twelve years and I love the land and its people, but also because along with many others, I believe New Zealand has the potential to become a role model for the world as a peaceful, sustainable, forward looking, and multicultural nation.

Aotearoa - New Zealand, the *Land of the Awakening Dawn,* is natural for this role. It has a small population, geographical isolation, natural beauty and resources, indigenous wisdom, a politically indepen-dent stance on global issues such as nuclear energy, and a practical pioneering mindset. The land abounds with practical dreamers and it is easy to connect with like-minded people here. As an immigrant from the UK, I have been uplifted by a sense of hope for the future which sadly, was more difficult to find in the more densely populated land of my birth.

In this book, I will introduce you to some of the little known but extraordinary people who are "living their passion as Love-in-action" in New Zealand. I hope these people will inspire you, as they have me. I see them as harbingers of a new culture, living at the unfolding edge of social change. They are developing life enhancing social innovations alongside the old, unsustainable ways. Each one holds a different strand of a new cultural weaving and is totally committed to making her or his own unique contribution, whilst they build community together, and in their own spheres of influence. As the book unfolded, I came to see them as evolutionary seeds of a new culture, germinating new social patterns and cultural models for a whole new future for humanity and for life on Earth.

I believe this group of people offers a rich soulful spread of ways of being, doing and thinking, and I hope there is something here for every reader. Whether you are a teenager trying to make sense of the world, a CEO of a large company, someone who's interested in living in intentional community, a local government policy maker, a teacher, or whoever you are, I hope you will find something in these pages to inspire you to be more courageous in your pursuit of a fully lived life, and to make you think more deeply about the world we share and how you can contribute to making it a better place for everyone.

## New Zealand's bounty

When I first arrived in New Zealand I was on a quest, although I wasn't fully aware of what I was looking for until I found it. I had decided to follow my creative process wherever it led me and had made a commitment to discover what it means to live consciously. I was also searching for a more soul-oriented life. I found more than I'd imagined possible: a safe haven amidst natural beauty where I could realize and deepen my connection with the essential Self; spiritual communities in which I could discover, explore, and expand my understandings of consciousness, soul and spirit; and a deeper purpose in life through working with others to bring positive change into our troubled world. In part this book is an act of gratitude for the bounty I have received.

Within a few months of my arrival in Aotearoa, I met two renowned New Zealand teachers who helped to shape my picture of this land. The first was Barry Brailsford, historian, archaeologist and author. I arrived shortly after he published his beautiful book, *"Song of Waitaha"*. He wrote about three races of people: the black, the brown, and the white people, who migrated to Aotearoa in their waka and lived together in the ways of peace for one thousand years, building a nation founded on peace. I know this has been a controversial book and I cannot tell you whether it is factually true or not. Yet the story of a nation of people living in the ways of peace for one thousand years is deeply inspiring to me. Barry speaks of the power of stories in people's lives and how we need new stories to unite us and remind us of our place in the cosmos and our connection with the natural world. The story of a People of Peace resonates with an eternal truth, pointing both backwards and forwards. It touches a deep longing to connect and become the One-Hearted-People. In my own heart, I identified as one of the People of Peace, and my arrival at the top of the South Island of New Zealand, where I decided to settle, felt like a homecoming. Such deep intuitive feelings are a resonance of the soul and cannot be explained. It is on this level I understand Barry's work. He introduced me to a land rich in mythology and vibrant with soul. When I embarked on a Peace Walk around the South Island, we carried a beautiful piece of pounamu, or greenstone, gifted by Barry. I learned it is a heart stone, sacred to Maori. I wear a piece around my neck as I write. Wherever I am in the world, it connects me with Aotearoa.

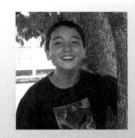

*Yaser: An All Rounder Seed*

My WHOLE NEW WORLD seed would be an all rounder seed because when you plant it, it will instantly grow into a row of happiness and give out fruit and love to the world. My planet would be a planet of rivers and unharmful creatures. I would send one or two countries that are allies and produce no pollution and nuclear power plants to grow the first seed.

The second teacher who influenced me was Dr Rangimarae Turuku Rose Pere, Maori spiritual teacher and leader. She spoke of Aotearoa as a retreat centre for the world, a place where people "come to find the lost pieces of their soul". She cautioned, once we have found our lost pieces, we must go out again into the world, taking our wisdom with us, to help heal the world. This book is my way of taking some soulful learning and New Zealand wisdom into the world.

New Zealand is a land which supports people's quest for deeper purpose, and I had only been in the country two months, when I received a vision for my soul work: to create a Holistic Learning Centre. At that time I wasn't ready to take action on this mission, so I put it on the back burner. Over the next ten years I brought the vision forward every so often and extended it. By 2001 it had become a vision, which I know is shared by others, for a Transformational Learning Centre, a place where people could gather from around the globe, to discover and practice the skills we need to carry us safely through this time of global transition. Last year, in 2006, it became clear to me New Zealand doesn't need a Transformational Learning Centre because it already *is* one! I felt I could make a contribution by connecting people, who are working within leading edge projects throughout New Zealand, into a community for transformational learning. As a lifelong educator and bodhisattva-in-training, I am interested in identifying the skills, values and processes emerging through this transformational work, and passing them on to support the acceleration of the collective process.

Through connection with an educational colleague in England, Bryce Taylor, I was introduced to the concept of globally responsible leadership. On a mission to find others who resonated with this concept, I met Daring Donna and began to participate in the network of Co-Creators in Auckland, where I witnessed the seeding of many transformational projects. Buoyed up by the upbeat energy of co-creation, I realized the time of change so many of us have been waiting for is upon us! Within this exhilarating movement of conscious evolution, I have chosen to live my lifelong passion as a writer, to gather some of the evolutionary seeds and spread them abroad!

## *Laying the tracks*

This book explores the notion of what it means to live one's passion by being Love-in-action. I have come to see this as a process of initiating creative actions which serve, conserve, and extend the well-being of the whole; a journey of experiential learning through which we develop consciousness and community. Amongst the passionate innovators I know, some are visionaries and writers holding a vision for the new to come whilst many work to develop community, make corporate environments more people-friendly, or create new models of business. Others are working to ensure basic life supports are maintained by, for example, contributing to the conservation of the world's diversity of fruit and vegetables, through seed saving, before the seeds are lost through the extinction of honey-bees, contact with genetically modified genes, or other toxic environments. There are people practicing natural methods of farming such as permaculture. Others are focusing on low impact housing and co-operative living in eco-villages; harnessing solar and wind power; saving water through composting toilets. There are healers of all descriptions assisting others to release blocked physical, emotional, and psychological energy, or teaching optimum well-being through the life-giving properties of raw foods. There are those working with teenagers to give them empowering opportunities for rites of passage. Some, within existing health services, are bringing multidisciplinary teams together to create more holistic provision for children, or teaching compassionate communication skills as an alternative to domestic violence. Some are bringing more understanding into the process of death and dying, whilst others are demystifying the global monetary system and creating community currencies as an alternative.

## Innovative Projects

One of my desires in writing this book is to share some of the exciting, innovative, grassroots projects which are transforming local communities. I first met Margaret Jefferies in the late 90's, when she was launching her first "Spirit at Work" conference and courageously giving voice to her own vision for New Zealand. Now she is working to bring vitality into her home community of Lyttelton, on the outskirts of Christchurch, doing inspirational role modeling for grassroots community development. At the year 2000 Heart Politics gathering, I met Robin Allison and heard about her vision for "Earthsong", an eco-neighbourhood in the suburbs of Auckland. When I interviewed her, she was in the final stages of the project, nearing the end of a thirteen year journey with it. Through the Co-Creators network, I heard about Leanne Holdsworth's Caring Communities Project, which raises community awareness within organisations and corporations, and James Samuel's vision for the localization of resources on Waiheke Island. Through networking to bring a Transformational Learning Community together, I connected with Vivienne Anne Wright and her brilliant global initiative, "One People One Planet", which aims to link school children around the world as "Peace Pals"; and with Kat Burns of "Positive Elements", a project creating a learning exchange with communities in developing countries.

## The journey of consciousness

What rings out clearly in all the interviews is that, at least as important as what we meaningfully do, is the quality of conscious being we bring to our endeavors. What characterizes and links the people within these pages is their commitment to conscious evolution: the realization all life is one interconnected, indivisible, evolving and participatory whole. This understanding of the creative unity of life is called "spirituality". It is not a doctrine, creed, or religion. Rather, it is an experiential, subjective process; a journey which we each take alone, and which ultimately connects us all. We come to understand the inner world through developing awareness and reflecting on our own experience and an important part of this journey is learning to give expression to our own authentic truth and creativity.

Finding a language for our perceptions, intuitions and realizations, and communicating with others with the intention of finding shared meanings, contribute to the development of a new culture, which includes the inner life, and creates a world with depth and dimension. These interviews include some deep personal sharing: I have spent my lifetime exploring the creative process as a writer, educator and Gestalt therapist, and I am particularly interested in the deeply redemptive aspect of inner work. Jonathan Evatt explores the creative process as universal power challenging personal power to come into embodiment. John Massey, healer, gardener and yoga teacher, reflects here on how stillness and observation contribute to our realization of the oneness of life, and how difficult it is for most of us to come to a place of stillness so we can make this connection. Mirjam Busch and Rudolf Jarosewitsch are psychotherapists who have been focusing their work on conscious relationship and compassionate communication. They now find themselves in a new, unknown "space" and challenged by the process of differentiation. Anahata and Orah Ishaya talk about their journeys toward unity consciousness through their work as spiritual teachers and healers.

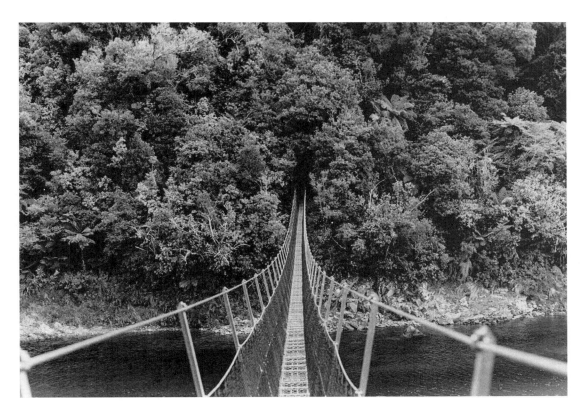

## Our relationship with nature

Alongside the recognition that humanity is one interconnected global family, arises the realization we are responsible for conserving and replenishing our environment. Just as our separation from each other is a tragic misperception, so too is our alienation from nature. Frank Cook is passionate about the healing power of plants and simple living. David Dwyer was setting off on a new adventure to establish permaculture in Golden Bay, when I spoke with him. He talked eloquently about the communion he feels with nature and the crisis he was thrown into as a teenager when he realized the social system he was being educated into is destroying the natural world he loves. Robina McCurdy, one of the founding members of the beautiful Tui Community and a lifelong educator and community builder, talked to me about a transformational learning project she created with her partner, Huckleberry, to build their home by the principles of earth-building and deep sustainability.

## Culture making

Having explored the theme of "Living your passion" through many rich interviews, I next asked the questions: what kind of new culture will grow from the evolutionary seeds of these people, ideas and projects? And how is a new culture actually created? Chris and Takawai Murphy talked to me about their work in race relations and their wonderful nationhood building course, Pumaoamo, reminding us how important it is to respect differences and diversity. They hold a vision for Maori and Pakeha New Zealanders to work side by side as partners, preserving their own ways, knowledge and languages. Jim Horton and Susan Jessie shared their experiences of living in intentional community, developing powerful men's and women's gatherings, and further extending this work to teenage girls and boys through their rites of passage programmes, Tides and Tracks. Their interview ends with a heartfelt call to value our boys and girls and empower them to make a positive transition to adulthood. For Vivienne Anne Wright the ultimate reason behind all our initiatives, as we transform communities, businesses and systems, and imbue them with the spirit of a new consciousness, is to ensure our children and grandchildren have a world fit to inhabit. We are the guardians of the world. Perhaps we need collective rites of passage to enable us to step into our responsibility!

## A new consciousness arising

The interviews in this book represent, for me, the spirit of unity in diversity. While each person makes a unique contribution, I was struck by the similarity of values. *How* we live our passion is an expression of our uniqueness and a contribution to diversity. *What unites us* is a vision for a new world arising from a new consciousness: the consciousness of our essential interconnectedness and co-creative potential..

In choosing contributors, I aimed for a balance between genders and a mix of people from both North and South Islands. Amongst those interviewed we have an age range from twenty-two to mid sixties, incorporating a broad range of interests. It seemed at first all contributors would be native New Zealanders, but as the book followed its own course, it embraced people from many lands. Some of the interviews are more conceptual, whilst others are in the form of more personal stories. In some, I had on my educator's hat and focused on particular interests such as leadership, or how to build a container for group alchemy. Originally, my intention was to write a series of short e-books based around the pillars of transformation: inner work, conscious relationship, living your passion, and co-creative community. However, when I reached my first fifty pages, both Donna and Woods told me they saw the potential for a full length book. I acquiesced, and from that point onwards, selected people according to the themes I wanted to develop, such as consciousness or culture making; or to create an age or gender balance. There are others I would have loved to include and, I was so uplifted by the interviews, I did not want to stop. This is a sampling, an appetizer and perhaps an example of a new genre: using interviews and conversations to capture the evolutionary flavour of this pivotal time in the history of humanity.

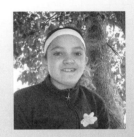

*Tyla: A Peace Seed*

My WHOLE NEW WORLD seed would be a peace seed. I would select this seed to stop all the fighting around the world. The peace seed would grow and all the fighting in the world would stop. All the children would get an education and the United States and Iraq will live in peace. My seed will grow into a world where everybody from different countries will be friends with each other.

## The children's seeds of peace

The idea to include seed thoughts from children came after the interview with Vivienne Wright. I wanted to give them the opportunity to add their own wonderful and refreshing wisdom. I asked the questions: if you could plant a seed for a whole new world what kind of seed would you plant? And what would your seed grow into? Vivienne kindly spoke with teachers from some of the schools she has been working with in Auckland and within a very tight time frame, children's words and photos were winging their way to me from Sunnybrae Normal School and Sherwood Primary School.

## A local/global vision

This book gives voice to a handful of passionate people working at the unfolding edge of social change. I see them as a fractal of a greater whole. During the course of writing I heard about a new book by Paul Hawken, *Blessed Unrest,* which confirmed my intuitive understanding there are millions of individuals and small organisations around the world working for positive change. And there are millions more ready to seize the opportunity for change if only they can be convinced a new way of living is possible. I am writing for all those who long for a new world and are ready to take the next step to becoming conscious creators of that new world.

Like many immigrants before me, when I first arrived in New Zealand thirteen years ago, I thought I had found Paradise, a dreaming place outside the mainstream. Over time I recognized my wishful thinking. There is no safe place to hide, nor is there any individual salvation. Wherever we are, we are part of One World. I echo Bob Harvey's question in the foreword, "What is this country capable of delivering?" What is New Zealand's unique contribution to the world in this time of global chaos? The people in this book offer a new, inspiring story for New Zealand, a song of hope. It's the story of a grassroots movement leading the way, and modeling to the world, the potential for people to live together in peace and harmony, with each other and with the land.

Peace begins with committed work within the self and extends into all relationships. This is no easy feat. Thousands of years of social conditioning cling to us in all sorts of gross and subtle ways, resisting our efforts at transformation. Yet this transformation is under way, and the fact that it is a grassroots movement makes my heart sing. At times when it seems everything is hanging by a thread, and the tissue of collective illusions which has held society together, seems gossamer fine, I remember there is a strength and power underlying everything. It is the strength of the people and the power of the land.

How will New Zealand step into its new story? I envision this grass-roots movement for cultural transformation being backed by policy decisions and resources; multi-faceted gatherings of innovative minds; a greater willingness on the part of policy makers to listen to what people want, need, long for, and are creating. My heartfelt prayer is that the beauty and soulfulness of Aotearoa, Land of the Awakening Dawn, will be preserved.

To embrace a global vision means making a shift of perspective from self interest to the highest good of all. New Zealand isn't the only country in the world with a new story to bring to life; each nation has its own unique contribution to make. And beyond national boundaries there is a new global story to co-create. There is a global network of conscious change-makers linking up now, creating what Teilhard de Chardin called the 'noosphere', a field of consciousness, or the thinking layer of the Earth. Back in the 1960's, he prophesied human life would become increasingly complex, and to balance the complexity, humanity would connect heart to heart, to experience itself as one body within a Whole Earth.

We have the opportunity to discover our unique life purpose or passion within a world evolving into one unified field of conscious-ness: one heart, one mind. What a magnificent gift! Creating a strong network to connect innovative evolutionary projects will support our understanding and accelerate shifts in consciousness. These in turn will transform personal lives and social institutions. Knowing there are many others working with the same values is encouraging. The web of Love-in-action around the world strengthens as we participate more fully in this planetary transformation from our own backyards.

Imagine a world in which every person is free to live their passion and offer their unique gifts into the co-creative weaving of the collec-tive life of humanity; a world in which passion and enthusiasm are encouraged. When work and livelihood are done in a spirit of love, integrity, and service, everyone benefits. This is how organic collective life works. When we offer our love and consciousness with true intent for the good of all, the Universe moves to support us.

I am heartened by the authenticity of the contributors in this book and have a burning desire to spread their sparks of passion and inspiration throughout New Zealand, and beyond. It's time! Consciousness is awakening! As Gandhi taught, we *are* the change we want to see in the world. All over the world positive, creative initiatives are pushing up from the grassroots; people are exercising their power and freedom; choosing to live in service to higher values and work together for the good of all. The world is becoming green with the vibrancy of new life. We inhabit a Mystery, much bigger than any mind can grasp.

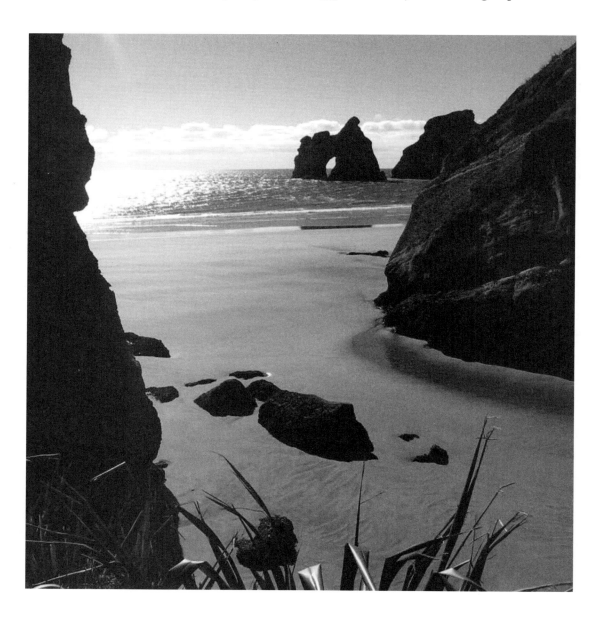

## Consciousness shifts are central to transformation

As the global deathing/birthing process deepens, people all over the world are experiencing an existential crisis. This is a crisis of perception and meaning. When we look at what is happening in the world we may be totally focused on the breakdown of systems, as in war, peak oil, famine, the thawing of the ice fields, the gap between rich and poor, and the extinction of species. In our personal lives, the crisis manifests as rising fuel and food bills, rising temperatures, deepening debt, less nature to play in and enjoy, working longer for less reward, the frustration of not being able to speak to a real person when we need service from the corporate world. Believing this is all there is evokes fear and leads to feelings of powerlessness, rage and depression. We all have our own ways to numb ourselves so we don't have to feel our fear and despair, but such numbing also robs us of joy, liveliness and motivation: the fuel for living our passion.

Glimpses of a more harmonious, purposeful universe can lead to an awakening of consciousness and a search for a deeper purpose to life. Becoming disillusioned with the ways working and social life are organized, may lead to a longing to break out and find something more satisfying, or to a desire to pursue and express one's creativity in a more specific way. Thus we may turn away from the life that is limiting our potential, to learn the skills of living our passion.

Consciousness develops through a number of shifts of perception, meaning and behavior; some people call these epiphanies. Such shifts happen instantaneously and reconfigure our perception of reality in a whole new pattern or gestalt. The perceptual shift is accompanied by an energetic shift, as energy is freed from old conditioning and 'stuck' forms. We sense a lightness of being, a coming home in some way, and a new feeling of empowerment.

Ah-ha! Looking at human interactions from a different angle, we suddenly see the growing number of individuals and groups who are working to create a positive future, like a host of little green shoots pushing up from the ashes of the old ways. Maybe a new world is possible after all!

Birth is a messy and frequently painful affair. This is a chaotic time which calls out the unlived potential in all of us. The process of becoming Love-in-action: authentic, creatively empowered and globally responsible, is a journey of experiential learning, leading to greater trust and awareness. This process enables the development of the skills and wisdom necessary to be of service to humanity and evolves through a series of transformational shifts.

# Transformational Shifts to the NEW CULTURE

* The shift from seeking satisfaction outside ourselves, to an exploration of inner being and inter-being through a process of experiential learning.

* The shift from head to heart; from fear to love, and ultimately to whole mind.

* The shift from feeling trapped by circumstances, to recognition that life is a journey of courage, trust and discovery, and we are creators capable of making conscious choices.

* The choice to withdraw our energy from what is not working and instead put our attention on what we choose to create.

* The shift from relying on outer authorities, to connecting instead with inner guidance, authentic values and creativity.

* A shift in identity occurs when we recognize we are not our thoughts and commit to mastering our minds.

* The shift from self interest and exploitation, to the choice to live in harmony.

* The shift from an illusion of separation and a belief that we have to "do it alone", to the realization we are participants in an intelligent, abundant and friendly universe, which is calling us to be of service to the whole.

* The shift from feeling separate, to building sustainable, co-creative community, wherever we happen to be.

* The shift from businesses which create huge profits for a few, whilst destroying the environment, to new sustainable models of business which honour life and give back to communities.

* The shift from concepts of "mine" and "yours" to recognizing the Universe is a constant flow of energy, and giving and receiving are one.

* The shift to the realization of Unity.

# THE INTERVIEWS

## The Journey

# *Shift One*

## From seeking satisfaction outside ourselves, to an exploration of inner being and inter-being through a process of experiential learning.

Courageously following the call of the heart to discover one's authentic being, is a healing journey into the unknown depths of self. Experiential learning is the process of expanding awareness, self knowledge, and self responsibility, through action, reflection, experimentation, honest communication and feedback. Rather than being solely focused on achieving goals and outcomes in the outer world, the process of learning becomes a primary source of meaning in life and the journey itself becomes the goal.

Living our passion is a journey through which we unfold our creative potential. The participants in this book all use slightly different language to describe their journey. Some call it a journey of consciousness; others speak of the soul journey, or walking an authentic spiritual path. My own journey has progressed through a series of leaps into the unknown, motivated by a strong desire to extend and actualize myself, to make my own unique contribution. To me, this is the most fascinating aspect of human life. Like the spider who weaves a web from her body, we make our life force available to bring something into being that didn't exist before. The power of the creative urge frequently imbues this wondrous process with a sense of inevitability, choicelessness, or destiny at work.

At the same time, if we want to create an authentic life, we must consciously choose it and activate our creative powers, not simply sit and wait for it to unfold. This choice sets us free to discover our own unique gifts and calling, and leads us away from blind conformity to societal expectations. For most people, the process of becoming authentic unfolds over many years and evolves through shedding and redefinition, accompanied by a growing awareness of spirituality, and a deepening connection with the essence of who we truly are, which is the same essence in every other being.

This is a journey of experiential learning focused on the creative process itself. As we are moved to creative action, we shift into new and deeper dimensions of being and discover who we are in this new territory, and what lies inside us awaiting expression. It becomes clear, creative thought and creative impulses originate in something much greater than our own individual mind or will. We are in some mysterious way connected both with a collective consciousness and with an originating force.

Moving from the known, whether this is leaving the familiarity of family, country of origin, or a career path, and stepping into the unknown, requires us to learn to trust life in a more radical way. We learn to trust our "inner voice": intuition and the longings of the heart. This moves us towards our "soul work": work that is uniquely ours to do, which will stretch and expand us, and lead to self healing.

It is not our actions alone which contribute to the common good, but our states of being or consciousness. As we undertake our soul work, we learn to trust in our own resources, or in our ability to connect with Source and re-Source ourselves from within. What is Source? In this book I refer to it as the universal intelligence that flows through everything, the evolutionary force, the divine spark in each one of us. This is the essential Self which is the goal of every spiritual path. The unconditioned, pristine, timeless centre of Being; pure love and creative potential, connecting us into One Life and One Heart.

Some of us listen to this evolutionary intelligence, others feel or sense it, for some it appears as images or visions. Sometimes this in-formation comes knocking on our door so loudly, we can't ignore it. We learn we are in co-creative relationship with this universal intelligence. We learn to be receptive to it and curious about it. We discover how to ask for guidance, how to wait and how to focus; how to hold an intention whilst at the same time being open, flexible, and unattached to outcomes. We learn to trust something broader than the rational mind and to value something deeper than the personality. We discover we are more than we ever thought we were. Yet at the same time, we lose some of our grandiosity and pride.

# INTRODUCTORY INTERVIEW
# WITH THE AUTHOR

## *Rose Diamond with Woods Elliott*
## Soul work, the creative process in action.

**Rose Diamond:** All her life, Rose has been asking the questions: "What does it mean to be alive on Earth at this time? What am I really here to do? What unique contribution can I make?" The answers have come as she chose to uncompromisingly follow her creative process and live her life as a journey of experiential learning. A lifelong educator and visionary thinker, she has spent much of her life in groups: educational, therapeutic, spiritual and dialogic. An avid reader, she early developed theoretical and practical interests in psyche, culture and the process of liberation. A compulsion to write started in childhood and developed through a mix of inspiration, perseverance, experimentation, and a burning desire to understand and communicate her experiences. A passionate love of wild nature has led her to seek sanctuary in beautiful places and fired her commitment to social transformation. Born in England, she lived nineteen years in Scotland before leaving in the early '90's to begin the soul journey which brought her to Aotearoa - New Zealand in late '94. She made her home in Nelson and Golden Bay at the top of the South Island, where she wrote and published her book: *Migration to the Heartland: a Soul Journey*

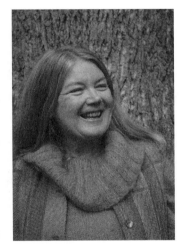

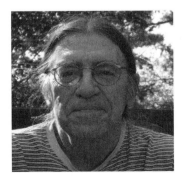

*in Aotearoa.* New Zealand has been a place of spiritual deep-ening and community participation for Rose. It is a natural Soul Sanctuary she longs to see preserved as a place of inspi-ration and solace for its people and for the world. Her dream is to create a sanctuary for deep soul work in Golden Bay. **www.soulsanctuary.co.nz**

**Woods Elliott:** Born in the US, Woods studied philosophy and art in college and earned a master's degree in social work in '69, pursuing a fifteen year career in the mental health field in psychiatric, child abuse, relationship counselling, family therapy, and correctional settings. Conscientious objector during the Vietnam War, civil rights and mental patient activist, great admirer of Native Americans. By the late '70's, he couldn't contain a midlife push for fresh adventures, and migrated to the Rocky Mountains in Colorado. Here he taught himself home-based furniture restoration skills and had a love affair with Mother Nature that stirred him into environmental activism, prospecting for gold and Indian artifacts, and culti-vating an alternate lifestyle. Open heart surgery at age 49 opened his heart in more ways than one and cast him onto a more spiritual path. Daily meditator, lifelong ponderer, unpub-lished writer, and enthusiast of Eckhart Tolle, Rose Diamond, and New Zealand, Woods would love to see New Zealand birth a new spirit and nature-centred society and eventually a whole new world. **www.awholenewworld.net**

**Woods:** As the author of "*Living your Passion*", Rose, what does it mean to *you* to live your passion?

**Rose:** When I look back over my life, I realize my main fascination has been the creative process itself and the unfolding of that, going into my own process and discovering what it means and how it works. At the core of living my passion is the ideal of living an authentic life; a life lived from my own creative centre. Although I didn't start out with this in mind, it appears my life has unfolded, and is unfolding, in a way to provide me with the experiences I need, to learn to live authentically, express myself fully, and be of service.

It started for me in 1983, when I left a fulltime job in adult education. My ostensible reason for leaving was to give myself time to write. I was working on a long, mythical poem which was the beginning of my exploration of soul, and I was experiencing a lot of tension between the educational work which I loved and the intense excitement of discovering the inner life for the first time. A whole new dimension of my being had opened up and it was very compelling.

Although I left my job in order to write, it didn't turn out like that! Instead, I started working freelance as a personal and professional development trainer and went on to create my own business. I'd already developed a taste for initiating projects and taking them from seed idea into action research and written materials. I was supporting developments in informal community learning, particularly in women's empowerment, and providing skills in communication and group leadership. My passion for this work made me fearless at some level.

## *Time for being*

When I took the leap from the security of the monthly pay cheque, I had to learn how to steer my own course according to the requirements of my own creative process, and support myself financially at the same time. I had a lot to learn! It's been a challenging, evolving process ever since and I love the freedom of it. I'm highly self motivated and work much more creatively when I can choose my own hours and honour my "down" times as well as my highly productive times. Much as I loved my job, it wasn't just nine to five, it was nine to five plus evenings plus weekends, and that driven quality was accepted as normal. There was no room for just being. I started writing poetry and that became an absorbing, centering meditative practice which took me deeply into myself, providing the balance I needed. It gave me permission to sit for hours listening inwardly for the next line, much as a fisherman sits by the side of a river. Taking time for being, and honouring the cyclical nature of creativity, have become increasingly important to me over the years. Nature is cyclical, women's bodies are cyclical, and I believe the soul evolves through cycles. Whereas, I see much of conventional working life as being very time-bound and linear, and that creates stress and burn-out in people.

**Woods:** Are you saying that for you living your passion is somehow tied up with following your own creative path and rhythms?

## *Listening deeply*

**Rose:** That's right. At a certain point in my life I made a decision to follow my creative process wherever it led me. Paradoxically, it took me beyond self interest. I've always come back to writing at times when I've made the greatest leaps of transformation. Writing seems to be at the core of living my passion. It's a wonderful tool for exploring experience more deeply and I love the challenge of bringing something into form, especially something as complex as a book. One of the key skills of writing seems to me to be the ability to listen deeply and be receptive to what one "hears" or intuits. In the past, I've understood this as listening to my soul, a deeper, more expanded part of me than every day consciousness. Now, I'm more interested in the idea that what is being heard or intuited is universal intelligence or spirit, and that we are all part of some vast, interconnected field of consciousness. I think projects which are successful arise from a field of collective consciousness and it's possible to "tune in" at some level to what is emerging. Maybe, in more profound moments, writing is a meeting between universal intelligence, "spirit", and the unique unfolding of individuality, "soul", and that's why it's so fascinating and compelling. For me, writing has been, and is, one of the most satisfying experiences of life, and it's certainly very closely tied up with the development of an authentic path and an authentic voice; and with the process of integration, which is essential for spiritual development.

However, writing hasn't always come easily to me. I've had to work at it over many years. When inspiration's flowing, it can be very exciting. There's a feeling of being carried by the creative energy, and if you follow, it leads you into the unknown, into new territory. But a lot of the time, it requires plain hard work and gritty determination. Once you've received the inspiration, you have to find the best form to express it and that involves a different set of skills and much pruning and editing. If you're writing for a particular audience, you have to consider what might be the best way to communicate with them, to reach and touch them. It's complex, and there's always more to learn. At some level, there's always a feeling of futility in the venture of trying to find words for subjective and mysterious experiences, which really can't be captured in words; or, in this case, the futility of trying to express leading edge ideas which are emerging very fast into the collective consciousness. It's a humbling experience coming up against the limitations of words and ideas and forms, and yet being compelled to continue the attempt.

I think there's a sacrificial aspect to following one's passion too. The creative process is about bringing everything to essence, or as close to essence as one can, so anything which is not essential has to be let go. This leads to greater simplicity. It may be the simplicity of living with fewer possessions or less external "security". It can also be a simplicity which comes through a process of integrating what can be quite complex ideas or experiences into more inclusive wholes. So there's an emergence of greater complexity expressed as simplicity, or wholeness. I have a favourite quote from the philosopher Martin Buber. He talks about the challenge of finding the intrinsic form of a work and says, "It breaks, or it breaks me". There's a sense of being pushed to one's limits by a greater power and having to learn both the laws and the discipline of how to co-create with that. Part of that discipline is being willing to go beyond the "little me", the needs of the personality, self indulgences and attachments. It's a process of holding a very clear focus and surrendering at the same time. You have to care enough to be willing to put in considerable time and energy, and yet be unattached to outcomes and not take it all too personally. It's really an exercise in aligning the personality and ego with the soul's purpose, and the soul has very different values and priorities. Quite tricky! In this sense I think living one's passion is about being a creative artist, whether the work of "art" is one's own life, a community project, or in this case, writing a book.

Much of my life since that first leap has been a balancing act between this compelling call of the inner life and the necessity to participate in society; between writing as a tool of self exploration and writing as an educational medium. The inner work always feeds and supports the outer work, and vice versa.

## *The Soul Journey*

**Woods:** Before your migration to Aotearoa, were there other radical shifts for you?

**Rose:** The second leap I took in '91-'93, when I made the conscious decision to follow my creative process. It took me first to the North West Highlands of Scotland and then to New Zealand on a soul journey adventure, which has lasted for fourteen years, and is ongoing. I discovered that following my passion, or my creative process, means allowing my unique path to unfold and being willing to go with that, even when it seems totally irrational or doesn't make any sense in terms of material security. That's the inspirational phase of the process: you can flow with it as an inner journey from the safety of home and you can also follow it as a physical life adventure. This can feel very risky at times, whether the risk is leaving physical comfort behind, or dropping a belief system and finding oneself in the unknown. I've had to learn how to support myself through the fear. Moving through fear and becoming aware of resistances are probably at the heart of most consciousness practices.

Before I left Scotland for New Zealand, I wrote the first draft of a book called "*Women and the Creative Process*", which I'd like to finish some day. I came to Aotearoa, intending to stay for a few months then return to Scotland to participate in a new business, but like many others, I fell in love with New Zealand, and the South Island in particular, and that was that! After a few adventures I settled in Nelson and was offered a job teaching counselling theory and practice which was perfect for me at the time. The job enabled me to consolidate my psychotherapeutic experience, extend my teaching skills and make a contribution to the community. It supported me to get residency in New Zealand as well, and later a friend came along and helped me to buy a house, so I became quite settled for a few years! For me! *Laughter.*

**Woods:** Oh, I bet you leapt again before long!

**Rose:** Yep! My third leap was in 2004, when I left my teaching job. I loved teaching but I was experiencing a growing tension between my own values and desire to express myself authentically, and the values of the profession and institution I was working within, which felt more restrictive and rule bound each time the institution restructured in response to the economic squeeze. I also had a strong feeling there was something more for me to do. I was still nurturing the vision I'd received when I first arrived in New Zealand, to create a Transformational Learning Centre, and I wanted to give myself time and space to see if this was indeed to be my soul work. So I went to live in Golden Bay until a clear direction emerged.

## Beyond the story-of-me

**Woods:** As you're telling your story, I'm thinking what an important vehicle personal storytelling is, both for integrating experience and moving beyond "the story-of-me".

**Rose:** Absolutely! Story-telling is such a powerful tool in many ways. Many people in this book talk about the uncompromising nature of living one's passion, and it has felt like that for me too. Ultimately my highest value is to be free to explore and express my own experience and to understand what it really means to be a human being living at this moment in history. I've been freer than many people to do this as I have not had the responsibility of raising children to consider. Paradoxically, I've found the deeper I go into myself, the more I discover everyone else. I think 10% of self is our uniqueness and 90% is our common humanity. The more I really explore my experience and understand myself, the more I find my belonging with the rest of humanity. Then I have more compassion for the human condition and I accept and love myself in a healthy and empowering way too. In this way, I've learned there is no separation between what truly serves me and what serves the whole.

**Woods:** Sounds like an important realization: when we actualize ourselves, we make our most important contribution to humanity.

**Rose:** Yes, I think the challenge and the opportunity at this time, when so many social institutions are being deconstructed, or have become corrupted, is for each individual to find their own authentic truth. There's an increasing pressure to do that, and my sense is the pressure comes from the evolutionary impulse itself. Authenticity is really about finding our connection with the rest of humanity, with nature and with cosmos, through being aligned with our highest truth and our authentic power. In order to make the evolutionary leap which I believe is possible for humanity at this time, we first have to experience our connectedness fully. The beauty of it is, the more truly we express the self, the more we connect. As soon as we realize we are essentially interconnected with every other being, we don't have any other choice but to serve that interconnection. It becomes apparent we are not separate, and whatever we do, to or for another being, for good or ill, we also do, to or for our self. Ultimately there is only one Self, one consciousness. I'm moving from an intuitive understanding of this awesome truth, towards the experience of living it in every moment.

My retreat time in Golden Bay enabled me to do a lot of healing around that sense of separation from self, others, and nature, and this is an ongoing process for me. Being in a very beautiful natural environment really helped me. I believe it is exactly this healing from separation to which the evolutionary impulse is calling us. Whenever any one of us heals in this way, we contribute to raising the collective consciousness to a level which will support the survival of our species and life on the planet.

**Woods:** Witnessing our own personal stories more deeply can contribute to becoming more aware of our common human nature. Joseph Campbell and, more recently, Tom Atlee have written interesting ideas about how we can enrich our stories so as to experience life more fully.

**Rose:** Yes, I think storytelling helps in several ways. It enables us to fill in "holes" in our sense of self. I did a lot of healing work with soul friend, Maggie Holling, around aspects of our stories which had been deeply traumatic for us. In both cases, this trauma occurred at a time when we were experiencing major consciousness expansion, or spiritual initiation. We had no language to express our experience nor was there understanding or support in our environments. In my case this happened within a therapeutic context and was deeply confusing for me. The therapeutic model is based on the idea of pathology and is inadequate for an appreciation of spiritual experience. It was only later, when I read a book by Stan Grof called, *"Spiritual Emergency"*, I really understood what had occurred.

Back in the 80's, I felt very alone in my soul journey. I was aware there were other people out there somewhere, yet I felt I was walking in a fog, up a mountain. I had to keep going and all I could see was the next step. Maybe there were other people out there, but I wasn't sure. I'd come to a little oasis, and there would be people there, then I'd leave again and re-enter the fog. I felt very much an outsider and scared at times. I was moving further and further from the mainstream, out on a limb, and the only way I could understand my experience was by going inside me and reaching into the deep to bring back poetic images. I really didn't have any choice. Once it was happening I just had to go with it. There was something much more powerful than me at play.

So, personal stories, yes! They help us to know we are not alone. They help us find a common language, to make sense of our experience, to fill in holes in self and liberate power that's become blocked and repressed. Revisiting our own stories with greater awareness supports us to become more authentic. We can chew up the experience and get nourishment from those aspects we identify with as being true for us, and spit out those we feel alienated from: the societal messages and conditioning we've swallowed whole, or people's negative reactions to us. Having our stories witnessed by others is very empowering too. I've taken part in many heart-sharing circles in New Zealand, where you stand with a talking stick and tell stories from your life; then listen attentively to the stories of others. Wonderful experiences!

**Woods:** Back to your story! It sounds as though Golden Bay provided you with a particular healing environment which was just what you needed?

**Rose:** Yes, I was in my mid fifties when I stepped out of "a secure job" for the fourth time, sold my house, packed what I could in the car, and took off. One of the things I have had to learn over and over again is, when it comes to soul work, everything takes much longer than I expect! My transition time in Golden Bay lasted for nearly three years, which was very challenging financially since I was earning very little. Although I was frequently stressed by lack of money, I was so compelled by the soul work I was doing, I really didn't feel able to make different choices. It seemed I was doing exactly what was necessary. It was a time of learning to surrender, to let go, and trust in a more radical way.

Golden Bay is a natural soul sanctuary. Maori call it "the prow of the ship" and, on a psychic level, it did feel to me like living right on the edge of consciousness and heading off into the unknown. With all that sea and sky, it's very open to cosmos; a perfect place for deep inner work, writing, creating and visioning. There's a saying: "Where land meets the sea is the place where magic is wrought." The land of Golden Bay has a powerful healing energy, and I felt it pulling me into alignment with a deeper purpose. It no longer felt like "my" deeper purpose, but the deeper purpose of humanity, which I was being called to serve by living my passion. The evolutionary impulse is very demanding. When we're willing and open, it constantly takes us to our limits, and beyond. It's always demanding more from us.

Although it was a time of retreat, I wasn't idle. *Laughter.* I self published my book, "*Migration to the Heartland: a Soul Journey in Aotearoa*", in 2004. This was a very freeing thing to do, an act of passion. It's the story of my own soul journey and tells how I migrated from Scotland to Aotearoa-New Zealand in search of a more soulful life. I worked on the book over eight or nine years as I was living the story. With Maggie, I laid the foundations for creating a Soul Sanctuary in Golden Bay and for a Transformational Learning Community, as well as doing the personal healing while letting go of the past. I feel immensely privileged to have had that time in Golden Bay and very grateful to all the people who supported me in different ways. It's a place that feeds my soul very deeply and I am still holding the dream for creating a Soul Sanctuary there, where people can come for deep soul work. People's need to "retreat" in this way will become more common and pressing, as more and more people of all ages are drawn into spiritual practices and explorations of the inner life. We need safe havens to do the work of inner reconstruction and for holding dialogue circles and deeper conversations.

**Woods:** Are you implying there is a natural drive in humans to deepen our experience and ever transcend ourselves? Is a certain amount of suffering a prerequisite for inner expansion and personal growth?

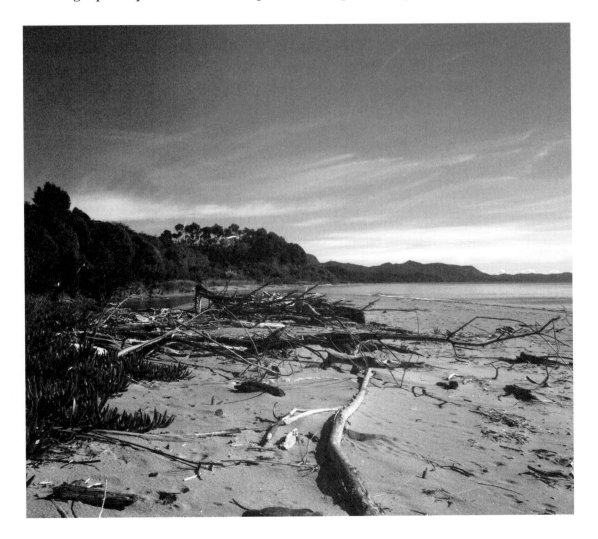

## *Death and rebirth*

**Rose:** There's a light and a dark side to living one's passion. The light side is about inspiration and being open to the cosmic mind, if you like. Both the far North West Highlands of Scotland, my first spiritual home, and Golden Bay, have elemental open landscapes with no obstacles in the way; very few distractions, and nothing external blocking communication from universal intelligence. That's the light part.

The dark part is the suffering involved. An elemental environment, with that sense of unrestricted freedom, brings me in touch with whatever is limiting me and separating me from my essential, loving nature. The search for the light, freedom, and love, inevitably brings to the surface whatever is not free, not light and unloving. In this way, I've been on a twenty or thirty year journey exploring the darkness in me, as well as the light. It's been very much about trusting I'm safe to go into the suffering and to allow whatever is arising to be healed. I find my strength in doing that. I surrender all the way to the bottom of the pain; I call it "bottoming out". I go deep, deep, deep into the well of self, and at the bottom, I often experience great weariness with life, a sense of loss or failure; all my beliefs appear to have been merely comforting illusions. If I stay with these feelings of despair and disillusionment and accept them, I'll find a new motivation to go on. I'll rise again, and be stronger for having risked the descent, and lighter for having seen through another illusion or false belief. It's a psychic death-rebirth process, which I call the way of the Deep Feminine.

This is one way I've received knowledge of the interconnectedness of all beings, and thus compassion, by going deep into pain and suffering and releasing the power that's been trapped by the conditioned mind. Whenever I've held back, or repressed my full self expression and passion in order to be accepted, or when I've been wounded in the attempt to fully express myself, some power has become trapped and unavailable to me. When I go into that deep place, it's not only my own pain and suffering I'm experiencing; it may be my mother's pain and suffering, women's pain and suffering, or humanity's pain and suffering. I see this descent into suffering and darkness, as a service to humanity. It's a different way of making a social contribution, not much understood in our culture. It's feared because people fear feeling their pain and often can't tolerate witnessing pain in another. We humans are such paradoxical beings; on the one hand, we're very small and puny in the scheme of things, but on the other hand, we are far more powerful than we allow ourselves to be.

My soul journey has been about living between the light and the dark, experiencing both, and learning to consciously choose the light, and take the next step towards it. We can't expand into the light and become more enlightened without also exploring the dark. When expansion happens, it's an overall expansion, high into cosmic freedom, deep into human suffering, wide into transpersonal love. It seems the very choice to live our passion brings us the challenge of facing and healing our pain and madness, and discovering compassion for the human condition. It is this combination of passion with compassion that creates Love-in-action or service. Without compassion, living one's passion can be merely self serving.

It takes an adventurous spirit to take these inner journeys. Writers throughout the ages have talked about love, creativity and madness being very closely aligned, and it can be crazy-making standing right at the edge of the unknown. But it's exhilarating also! Fear may pull us back from that edge into the more familiar apathy and hopelessness. It's important to discern when suffering is presenting an opportunity for healing and letting go of old stories, and when we're fearfully clinging to the familiarity of misery. Sometimes making the choice to be positive can be an avoidance of going deeper too. However, I think it's necessary to honour people's limits, everyone has the right to say, "this far and no further", although there's always a price to pay for that choice, as well.

I believe we all have the choice every moment of every day to choose life and love. We can choose to be more creative and more loving and support this choice through our daily consciousness practice. The more we make the simple choice to be creative and loving every day, the more the world becomes creative and loving. It sounds very simple, yet it is so difficult to do!

I'm at a point now where it all makes sense! The threads of my life are all woven together into a meaningful, beautiful tapestry. But that may change tomorrow as the next challenge arises! *Laughter.* These times of integration are like stepping stones or, maybe like the rings inside the trunk of a tree, they make the next expansion of consciousness possible. Sometimes on the path, it can be difficult to see where the successes are, because much of it is about letting go rather than adding something to self. Yet I have always trusted, and still do, that if I follow my excitement, I will be supported. And I have always been supported, even though I've taken risks and been down to my less than bottom dollar, I've been taken care of, always.

## *The making of "Living your Passion"*

**Woods:** It sounds as though choosing to pursue your soul work has led to a life of continuing adventure! Tell me how this book *"Living your Passion"* arose?

**Rose:** It's been very organic really. I wanted to use my skills and passion to inquire into the values, beliefs, and attitudes necessary to make the shifts of consciousness that will give rise to a new culture, and to use my writing skills to help catalyse that shift. I felt this would be the best way to give back the fruits of my experience and pull together the threads of my working life. I became very excited by the idea of drawing together the wisdom of some of the adventurous people I know in New Zealand who are working for the sort of social change I understand is needed. So one impulse behind this book was to provide a platform for people to stand up and be seen, to talk about what they're doing in their projects and say: this is what's happening, take notice!

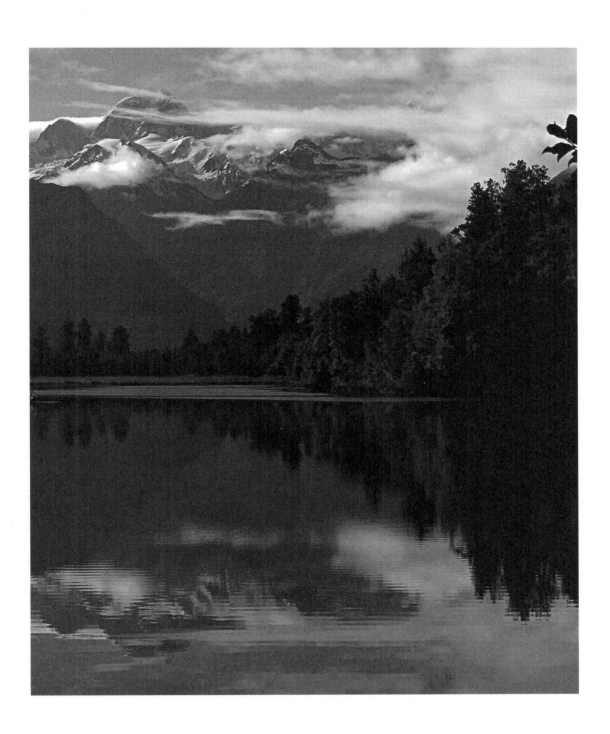

## *The magic of dialogue*

The book also takes up another life thread, a love of dialogue, and explores the potential of conversation as a creative medium. I came upon my love of dialogue originally through immersion in Gestalt therapy. For ten years, I took part in powerful experiential learning communities, as a trainee and therapist, and I worked for another ten years as a teacher of Gestalt skills. Unlike many therapies, Gestalt doesn't focus on problems, but on developing awareness of the creative process itself. Presence and awareness can give rise to the kind of transformational shifts, or ah-ha moments talked about in this book, enable us to step out of old patterns, and experiment with new solutions. Writing is one way of exploring the creative process, mostly a solitary way. Exploring the creative process with another person through dialogue is an act of co-creation. In a dialogue, you set off into the unknown, you're going somewhere and you don't really know where you're going! I find I'm saying things I didn't know I was going to say or didn't even know I knew! The conversation starts here and ends up somewhere over there! How we got there has been a mysterious unfolding! The skill is to stay very present at that place of unfolding. I love that, and right now, I'm returning to using that particular skill to help other people unfold their creative process more quickly, not as a form of therapy, but simply as a creative exploration of presence and living at the unfolding edge of experience, which for me is one of the most exciting things in life. Dialogue's a mutual interest that's brought you and me together Woods, in our exploration of conscious relationship.

## *The emerging culture*

**Woods:** In the interviews, you talk with individuals and couples who are "living their passion" and it quickly becomes apparent these innovative people represent a new, emerging culture, as I understand it. I find that exciting to say! We can give birth to what is needed! It's a departure from the idea of culture and counterculture, which is polarised and limiting. This, on the other hand, distinguishes itself as representing a fresh attempt to co-create a new, transcendent culture based on the common good.

**Rose:** Yes. One thing that characterizes these people I've chosen to interview is that they're not putting energy into resisting the dominant culture, or being angry. In the past, much countercultural activity was motivated at least in part by anger: civil rights, feminism, and the environmental movement, for example. Maybe anger was an appropriate motivating force for the time and certainly a lot of important evolutionary work was accomplished. Now there's a new consciousness arising and the recognition, if we put anger out into the world, we're contributing to the problem rather than creating a solution. Anger is always against something, so it increases the sense of "us" and "them", or "I'm right and you're wrong", power-over, polarisation, duality and separation. The new consciousness is more concerned with connection and understanding between people. It's inquiring, curious and inclusive, rather than reactive. It gives rise to a global vision, based on the philosophy and practice of being Love-in-action, being in service to the greater whole. This will lead in time to a state of unity between people. The pioneers of this emerging culture, of which people in this book are examples, all know what's going on in the world, but they've withdrawn their energy from what's not working, and they're completely committed to creating what they see to be the next necessary step towards a more humane world. It's a complete turnaround. I experienced it myself this last year. There's a point at which the pull of fear no longer holds you, and you stop doubting what you're doing, or whether you can do it. You stop resisting or fighting against something, and simply stand in the present, fully committed to creating the future. We're saying, ok, we're building a new culture alongside the old, and whoever feels attracted please join in. Whatever's happening elsewhere, this is what we're doing, and this is what we value.

**Woods:** So the new culture has new values to rally around rather than old values to quarrel over. Maybe you could tell us what some of these values are?

**Rose:** There's a realization that if we're going to survive as a species, we can no longer go along with the cult of the individual: me, mine, me first, me *or* you, me *over* you. We come to realize all life is sacred and connected and we take responsibility for that. I think that's the biggest shift. Creating community also becomes central if we want to survive into the future. Our basic resources like water, the quality of air we breathe, our sources of power, are all threatened as a result of the reckless ways we have been exploiting the planet. We need to learn to work together and be collectively responsible for decisions which affect us all, and future generations, rather than leaving such decisions to be made by a few people with vested interests, whilst the rest of us stand helplessly by. As we create conscious community, we can share resources and find solutions to common problems by evolving our thinking together. We can create far more magnificently together than we ever can alone. A willingness to drop our fears and step into inventive co-creative partnerships and alliances is the only way we are going to survive.

**Woods:** It's a shift from the individual freedom to take ourselves where we want, to pursue our latest 'thing' and be concerned with our own achievements in life, to this more community-centered kind of society. Sounds like an enormous shift requiring some amazing changes from us!

**Rose:** It *is* a big shift! The paradox is, although it requires us to give up some old habits, we gain <u>so</u> much. Living our passion, doing the soul work we're each uniquely here to do, leads to a discovery of increased abundance and prosperity, which isn't necessarily linked to money, although it may be. Money is a form of energy and exchange, which unfortunately has attracted many of humanity's most selfish and aggressive drives, but it can also create great good. Maybe this is the point in history when we need to free money from being "the root of all evil" and liberate it as a resource for the common good.

**Woods:** In America, I can imagine a difficult transition, because this has been a nation in which individuals are relatively free to pursue their own private goals unimpeded and irrespective of the common good.

**Rose:** I guess the United States represents the extreme of the Western lifestyle, and these beliefs about individual freedom being tied up with material riches, are deeply ingrained. My understanding is, people are usually ready to change when they're really hurting, and I think many people are hurting, as a result of the emptiness of the materialistic lifestyle. The trap of materialism is, we want something and then we get it, but the "getting" satisfaction is short-lived and we want a next thing, and so we get that. It's a never ending hunger, because what most people really want are inner peace and a sense of fulfillment, and these can only be found inside us, and then offered in relationship to others or in service to life. One of the things I've realized is, although people may feel dissatisfied and wish to change, they often don't know how, or there are no models to aspire to. This was definitely a motivation for this book; the desire to inspire people to actualize themselves, to spread the seed thoughts that we each make a difference and world peace begins in each one of us; and to fan the flames of a new dream for humanity. People will take the risk to make changes when they see something more sustainable and more nourishing is actually possible. Without new models, people won't be motivated. They'll keep doing what they've always done, because they don't know what else to do. These stories in *"Living Your Passion"* show us how we <u>can</u> change.

**Woods:** It's a radical departure from the old ways. We're often somewhat limited in our views, stuck in the reality of what exists, and the best we can do is slightly improve the mess rather than do something which allows us to depart from what exists, and thus transform it.

**Rose:** We're in a transition time. It takes commitment and a shift in priorities but these happen naturally when we discover what we're really here to do! There's a lot of foundation building to be done in the transitional phase, and important skills to be learned. For example, several people in this book talk about conscious relationship or compassionate communication. Most of us are beginners when it comes to these skills. Similarly, we're all learning about our own unique creative process, about the laws of manifestation and how to co-create. We're learning how to find a common language for our inner experience so we can support ourselves and each other through challenging times. We're learning how to live in physical, mental, emotional and spiritual balance as a day to day, moment to moment practice. We're learning how to be in dialogue with each other and to enter the unknown with open minds and hearts. We're learning to love consciously. To reach a new place and create a new culture require trust and faith along with dialogue and experimentation. At this point, this is not for everybody, but there are growing numbers of people leading the way. Partly, it's altruistic and partly, it gives the greatest personal satisfaction. That's the beauty of it. It isn't *either* I do something for myself *or* I do something for the collective. Most people in this book said: "I'm living my passion because I don't want to compromise. I'm doing this because it allows me to fully express myself by serving and giving my gifts."

**Woods:** I see the special folks in your book as living examples of the new paradigm. It seems to start with the individual and lead to recognition of the need for a new kind of consciousness and a new kind of community. Our problems are so sewn together we can't support these individual-centered cultures any longer. We need a society that balances self and other, and integrates the individual with an equally important communal and collective life. Somehow I've never quite looked at it this way before. Normally, we sort of inherit societal ways of doing things and find a nook within the social fabric. The notion we're here to evolve new societal forms rather than stay stuck with what doesn't work is new and different. We don't really yet know how to do that. We're so used to falling back on the cultural givens, into which we're born, and being very defined and limited by its older structures, we embrace a lot of things we don't necessarily have to embrace, because we think we don't have a choice; all these things are already in place. What we actually need is a whole new wave of social arrangements that break us out of confinement to these older ways of doing things.

**Rose:** Yes. We also need new cultural stories. Just as we can do personal story work, so too nations need to get very clear what they identify with and what special gifts they have to offer, and then be willing to make the leap of transcending national interests and identity and joining a new global story. This doesn't mean giving up our differences, but embracing them.

Most people in these interviews have opted for lives of voluntary simplicity, choosing to live with less material possessions in favour of the "social capital" to be found in community, or the spiritual fulfillment in the practice of Love-in-action. From a certain vantage point, people may see living more simply as a demand for them to give up their freedom, comfort and security. In fact there's nothing lost in living simply except limiting habits of mind; beliefs we have to have things "our way", which create conflict and stress; and fears about giving up whatever we understand our identity to be. It *is* a shift in identity. It's not necessarily an easy process as long as we struggle and resist, but when we let go and surrender to it, it's very simple!

**Woods:** That's part of the notion of a new consciousness arising among us? This I know is very central to your thinking. I was taken with the shift from head to heart; new ways in which mind and heart can dance together; new forms of intuitive knowing that enable us to grasp the whole of things: these seem to be parts of the new culture. You could call it "whole mindedness", an ability to integrate and synthesize disparate elements.

**Rose:** Yes, one of the things many of those interviewed say, each in his or her own way, is that there's a universal intelligence beyond the individual human mind, which is constantly evolving, and needs our participation to actualize itself. Inner listening is not just listening to our own psyches. We listen to the psyche in order to clear the mind and still the inner space, so we can bring the universal intelligence through. The more "little self" or "story-of-me" we can release through awareness and choice, the more easily we can receive this intelligence. That's the dance I see between the head and the heart. We bring our individual skills, life experience and wisdom, to this co-creation with universal intelligence. People who live this way are living on their own growing edge; on the edge between the known and the unknown. The less we are habit-bound, the more we can be open to the new consciousness coming through.

## *Making conscious choices*

**Woods:** I know partly you've been listening to these interviews with the ears of a passionate educator. You have a notion of a specific set of transformational skills or capabilities required for moving to a new culture?

**Rose:** Yes, there are many, but fundamentally it always comes back to our ability to make conscious choices in every moment.

**Woods:** Is this part of the new consciousness?

**Rose:** Absolutely. It's through our conscious choices we become agents in our own lives and agents of change. As long as we are able to see the choices we have, then we are free. We're not necessarily always free to choose what happens to us, but we're clearly free to choose how we respond to what happens.

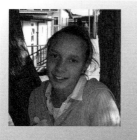

*Petra:*
*An Environment Seed*

*My WHOLE NEW WORLD seed would be an environment seed. It would grow into people looking after the environment, picking up rubbish, being happy and having fun.*

Undoing our conditioning requires a big commitment. It's not an easy thing to drop lifelong habits, but the rewards are great when we choose to step out of the old conditioned habits of mind and experience our essential authentic nature, which is always loving, harmonious, and creative. If you take someone like Eckhart Tolle, for example, who has become a hugely popular spiritual teacher; he lives these qualities of Love-in-action. He has a sense of humour and a wry irony about the way we live our life situations, but there's no malice there and no arrogance. He truly embodies the new consciousness.

**Woods:** I've heard you use the term conscious relationship many times. Is there some way in which the kinds of relationships we will have in the future are going to be different from those we now know?

**Rose:** Frank talks about how all his meetings were synchronous; Donna says welcome everybody; Rudolf and Mirjam talk about relationships as a healing path or soul journey. Practicing conscious relationship means seeing every single relationship as an opportunity to be Love-in-action. It's an opportunity to experience ourselves more fully and to see what blocks our creativity and love. Then we can choose to drop our old painful, limiting ways, see past the little self to our shared humanity, and serve that. Every relationship mirrors back to us whether we're in a state of love or in a state of fear.

There's a paradox that while we are essentially all One, we're all unique and different too, and that's what makes life interesting and a challenge! How can we relate to each other's differences without getting caught up in judgments, criticisms and comparisons? Can we really learn to tolerate and even celebrate our differences, rejoice in each other's achievements and encourage each other to 'go for it'? Can we support each other to be brilliantly creative and magnificent? It's quite tricky at times, because most of us in the West have been brought up in a competitive system, and envy will often creep in when someone does a great job or takes a leading role in life.

I believe every time one of us takes a step forward in consciousness, or steps out of a limiting pattern, it makes it easier for everyone else; there's more consciousness available in the environment. So for many of the younger generations, it's easier to be conscious than it was for us at, say, twenty or thirty. The new culture emerging now is evolving from the work of millions of people in the past. It's important to honour what has gone before, and to honour all the different current contributions as well. Innovations are never created by one person, but emerge from a collective consciousness when the time is right.

**Woods:** Do you think it's true some people are afraid to make transformational shifts, because somehow they feel they'll suffer more if they become more aware?

**Rose:** I think that's partly true. A great many people are anaesthetized. We all, to some extent, numb ourselves in order to cope with life. For example, when I really stop and feel my response to what's happening to the natural world, I feel an immense sadness. In order to live day to day and feel positive about life, I somehow tune out that sadness. I know very few people who don't in some way numb themselves, or rationalize away the complex feelings of living at this time. However to become more conscious requires us to experience and release our pain.

**Woods:** I suppose humans are so used to being in denial in order to cope with life's stresses, it's hard to convince them denying less and feeling more fully don't necessarily just raise the pain level. But facing fully what is, also leads to a new fullness of perspective, in which there's some liberation.

**Rose:** I guess that's why putting forward positive, life-enhancing examples, is a worthwhile thing to do, rather than focusing on pain and difficulty, which can keep us trapped. There's a delicate balance between being aware and not avoiding our pain, but not indulging it either. For some people, it's safer being in familiar pain than taking the risk of stepping into something new. Letting go of old patterns, the story-of-me, can cause fear, because when you let go of your story, who are you? It can be scary being in a new unknown place, feeling boundary-less, outside the comfort of habit, feeling a little lost and out-on-a-limb.

**Woods:** It seems so important to identify our resistances to becoming more fully conscious, and to be able to work through whatever scary aspects of change hold us back from more awareness.

**Rose:** Yes, being authentic means identifying with a deeper sense of self, coming to identify with the essential self which is universal, as well as with the little personality. We're all in the process of awakening. We can be awake one day and go back to sleep the next, and we are all at different stages of sleep or awakening. The positive aspect of our global crisis is an opportunity for humanity to awaken to what life can truly be, if we choose it. On the whole, humanity hasn't done such a great job on Earth, even though there are so many good people in the world. What's happening now is a wake-up call. I feel at a soul level, I've chosen to be here at this amazing time of choice. I don't claim to have the whole truth, but if I can make a difference by living my passion, then it's worth giving it my best shot!

**Woods:** Sounds like you have a vision for the future?

**Rose:** What has been spoken and written about in *"Living Your Passion"* is the beginning of a new future. People will live much more in community, developing local government through real dialogue, more like the Native American ways or the hui of the Maori; coming together in Sacred Space where everyone can speak, and everyone can be heard, and everyone is valued and accepted; and out of that truly democratic decisions are made. That's my idea of what a local government could be: real dialogue and consideration of the whole, rather than people protecting their vested interests at the expense of others, or at the expense of the environment. Community responsibility and participation are key elements; people coming out of their isolation and their little boxes; coming out of their fear and paranoia, to truly relate to each other and expand personal and collective empowerment. Margaret talks about small groups building community from the grassroots up, through practical innovations such as the farmers market. This creates real prosperity and abundance by increasing financial and social flow and putting more money in people's pockets. In this way people feel valued for their contributions, and relationships are formed and deepened. Leanne talks about extending this experience of community throughout the corporate world; fostering deeper understanding with policy makers about the daily reality of people's lives, and encouraging a more holistic approach to decision making, based on the values of social justice.

On the one hand, this process of changing consciousness appears to be linear and slow, taking place over many years. When I think of it like that, I can get a little blue about the future of humanity. I think perhaps we don't have time to make the necessary changes. On the other hand, transformation happens in an instant! When enough people shift into a higher state of consciousness or awakening, I believe we will collectively make a breakthrough. Anahata and Orah say it takes only 64,000 enlightened individuals to change the world by tipping the balance of consciousness into love and wisdom. Every individual can contribute to that collective consciousness shift. When you're with a group of positive, light-hearted people, it's easy to move faster; the synergy supports everyone to be their best. There is real power in linking up around the world. Paradoxically, we're involved in both a slow linear process of lifelong learning, whilst fast transformative leaps forward can also occur. We're definitely in a period of accelerated collective growth right now.

**Woods:** We need an "Up-wising", as the American comedian Swami Beyondananda puts it. *Laughter.* In my view, Rose, you have succeeded in these refreshing, novel interviews to suggest that the new culture is deeply infused with richer spiritual meaning, of which we've been so bereft in the old culture. That's so hopeful; as hopeful as the exquisitely soulful film, *"The Gathering"*, was for me!

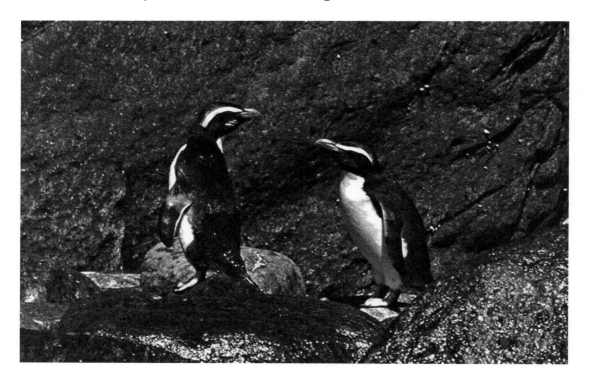

**Rose:** The new spirituality is very much about bringing spirit down to Earth; knowing everything is sacred and every individual being has a spark of the divine in them. We're living in, and are part of, an intelligent living system, and we can either impose our will on that, or we can listen to its intelligence and respond to it, participate with it, and bring our skills into play with it. It's a very exciting way of experiencing life. There have been groups of people throughout history who have held similar knowledge of a participatory universe: the Gnostics, the

Rosicrucians, and the Indigenous Peoples of the world, for example. It's just here we are again, ready to seize this present moment to bring Heaven to Earth. I truly believe humanity has been given a paradise to live in and we have surely messed it up, but perhaps that has been a necessary part of the evolutionary movement, to get us to this point from which we can make a collective transformational leap!

However differently people interpret what's happening, there can surely be no doubt in anyone's mind we're in a time of great change globally; change and upheaval of the physical world and all our institutions. I think something new and life-enhancing comes through only when enough people hold shared values and intention. We will have peace in the world when enough people really want peace so much we're willing to create it in our own minds and hearts, in our own relationships and families, and in our work teams and communities. That's where it all starts. The projects we create are experiments and vehicles for the new consciousness. What matters is, we're aligned with values that support the whole and value the whole, and we ask important integral questions and inquire into those questions together. How can we all live together in peace? There are nearly 6.6 billion of us on the planet right now! How can we feed, clothe, house and educate everybody? How can we conserve what's left of nature's bounty and beauty?

I look forward to watching the unfolding of events over the next few years and seeing New Zealand step up into its new story. Bob Harvey says in his foreword: "We can be teachers of wisdom, of mystery and of soul politics, of environmental truth and consciousness. We can wear the cloak of mana and carry the mantle of wise and good facilitators". Yes!

This book started as an exploration of innovative projects, but it's much bigger and more inspiring than that! It's actually about spirituality and making a commitment to a global vision and to unity consciousness. If we are to survive and thrive, we will move collectively to a more spiritual perspective; a perspective from which we can see we are all interconnected. We are all One.

# Finding a common language

We are at a point in our collective journey when growing numbers of people are finding a common language and common understandings for this experience of co-creation between our unique individual genius and the universal intelligence, or evolutionary impulse, which inspires our thoughts and moves us to act. I am struck by the similarity of experience amongst the contributors to this book. Will speaks of "a massive energy that consumes me and I don't have a choice." Kat talks about the unfolding of human potential in which, "I don't have a choice, it just happens." David speaks of "a real evolutionary process". Participating in this process evokes states of love, joy, freedom, harmony, excitement, simplicity, peace, and contentment. When we let go, trust, and flow with creative energy, we discover we are participating in an abundant playful world, full of synchronicities; a world which unfolds at our feet. David speaks of "being shown into a richer life". Frank says, "I do fully believe the Universe meets you." Kat says, "If you take that first step into the unknown, the Universe just picks you up and runs with you." There is a sense of connection and relationship, a mutual give and take, in which our needs are met when we live in trust.

Throughout human history, there have been people who journeyed into the Mystery of spirituality and mapped the territory for those who followed. Oftentimes such people were seen as a threat to those in power and were persecuted or silenced, as in the terrible holocaust of the European Reformation, when millions of innocent people were burned as witches, or the imprisonment of artists and poets under the Communist regime. At this time in history, there is a global spiritual renaissance happening alongside the chaos and deconstruction of old forms. As we are able to put words to our experience of expanding consciousness, and find a common language for it, the growth of collective consciousness accelerates exponentially.

These interviews put words to the journey and, although each one is unique and different, they reveal shared understandings of the process.

**Kat Burns** talks about living her passion as a path of joy and a return to the kind of simplicity she has discovered in developing countries. Kat is working with Positive Elements, a project with a global vision, which aims to unfold human potential, increase wealth within communities, and create a learning exchange between East and West. As a highly conscious twenty-six year old, Kat is discovering the skills of co-creative business and conscious relationship, as she learns to balance focus with flow within her own creative process.

**David Dwyer's** emphasis is on practical ways of living his spiritual ideals in communion with the Earth, through observing and co-creating with nature. For most of us, the journey to authenticity takes a long time, if we complete it at all, yet there are others who never seem to lose touch with their own truth and essential loving nature. Such beings exist in all generations and are often challenged by the restrictions of "normal life". David, aged twenty-two, is one of them. His conversation explores a crisis of values arising from a deep dissatisfaction with mainstream culture; often the starting place for the soul journey. He left me feeling optimistic, yet with some big questions about the loss of potential caused by an education system which focuses increasingly on training for employment rather than on drawing out the unique creative gifts of each individual.

**Will Lau:** When I first encountered Will at a Heart Politics gathering in January 2006, he had the serenity of a Buddha. It was only later I discovered he is a high powered, hi-tech entrepreneur. Will's story describes the process of doubt and breakthrough many people experience when they make the decision to leave a "secure" job and career path to follow their passion. A peaceful warrior, he has learned to turn his fear into an ally, which stretches him beyond his limits. He describes the leaps of trust required when the fire of creativity moves through him, motivating him to "punch through the fear". In a second shift of values, living his passion became Love-in-action, as he opened to spirituality, personal journeying, co-creation and service. He reminded me, the foundation for a new global culture has already been laid, through the World Wide Web of the Internet.

**Frank Cook:** Through his uncompromising commitment to authenticity and cultivating a simple lifestyle, Frank, an American, shows how opening to relationship with the natural world reveals the profound abundance and generosity of life; mostly forgotten in our busy, materialistic way of living. Frank showed up at Swanson Sanctuary at the end of a hitch-hiking tour of New Zealand, as part of his research into the plants of the world and what they have to teach us. Our relationship with nature is such an important aspect of the new consciousness, and my conversation with Frank was an inspiring reminder to slow down, be present, listen, and observe the natural world around us.

# What does living your passion mean to you?

*At the core of living my passion is the ideal of living an authentic life; a life lived from my own creative centre. My life has unfolded in such a way as to provide the experiences I need, to learn to live authentically, express myself fully, and be of service. —Rose*

*Living my passion is a feeling of joy in my heart. When I'm creating from a place of joy, I feel energy coming through me. True passion comes from a place of spirit. It's the path of most enjoyment, and if you follow that, you will be living your passion. —Kat*

*I recognize there's a sense of personal inner evolution, or inner self knowing, self realization I guess, and that's not dependent on any outer activity. It doesn't matter what I'm doing in the world, I feel at peace when I'm in touch with my true self and just by the nature of doing that, I'm sharing myself with the whole Universe and constantly becoming more blissful. —David*

*Living my passion is about having the courage to do what I really want to do in life. It's this massive energy that consumes me and I don't have a choice. Passion for me is a flame. The most passionate people tend to be really fiery. They get that flame and direct it, and look at what they're scared of, and just blow right through it, because it holds no power. —Will*

*Living my passion means not having to sacrifice or compromise myself to achieve my purpose here. For me it's definitely an everyday commitment. Every day for me, is about how many people I can talk to, share and communicate with. It's about getting people to wake up to where we really are. —Frank*

## We are transitioning through profound global change

Few people can be in doubt we are transitioning through profound global change. Every day we feel the effects of living at a time when the old ways of organizing our collective life are no longer working, whilst new ways are just beginning to emerge. Some see this as a time of breakdown, as old systems which have sustained life, crack under the strain of increasing complexity. Everything seems to be in need of a radical overhaul: the way we work, our relationship skills, even our sense of self, are all challenged by change.

From a certain perspective, humanity appears to be a species hell-bent on extinction; one of evolution's abundant experimental life forms failing to adapt. In the world at large, war, terrorism, the widening gap between rich and poor, peak oil, the environmental crisis of climate change and global warming, all contribute to a sense that we can no longer continue to live in the way to which we've become accustomed. All the signs are telling us: if we don't want to perish, we must change. If we want to thrive, we must create something entirely new.

Alongside our collective lack of wisdom, humanity possesses great creative brilliance, and the technological prowess we need to move into a new stage of evolution. We are a species which, when faced with the possibility of our own extinction, has the choice to evolve consciously. My hope is our current global crisis is providing just the right motivation in enough people, to bring about the shifts of consciousness required, to transform ourselves into a compassionate, globally responsible society, which values life and respects differences.

# *Shift Two*

## From the head to the heart; from fear to love, and ultimately to whole mind.

The journey from the head to the heart involves remembering who we truly are. At certain times in life, the heart feels the tug of the soul and hears the call to authenticity. When we choose to accept and respond to this call, we begin the journey to greater awareness and heightened consciousness. We achieve our ultimate power and creativity when heart and mind are in balance, working together in harmony, and able to synthesize diverse elements into more inclusive wholes.

# *Kat Burns*

## Get out of the way and
## let it all flow through you.

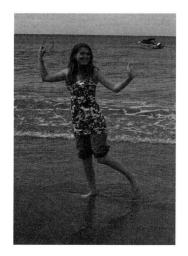

Kat Burns is a stubborn idealist and change-maker. Growing up with a strange sense of what the ** are we doing on this planet, she began searching for her place in it with a vague and persistent knowing things could somehow be so much better. Looking to make a contribution, she tried numerous studies, roles and travels, and finally, resorting to self-exploration, realized this is where the answer lies. She is passionate about bringing spirit into society, particularly business and social development, and creating spaces where people can come together in community to remember their true selves and oneness with each other and the planet. She is now co-creating a conscious business, Positive Elements, which creates wealth and opportunities for co-operatives and villages by promoting their sustainable handcrafts. Her dream is to co-create a network of communities around the world which support each other to realize their full potential and spread the message of our common unity.

**Kat:** Living my passion is a feeling of joy in my heart. When I'm creating from a place of joy, I feel energy coming through me. It's not something I decide I want to do from a mental level, "Oh, I think I'm passionate about that! I'm going to try that for a while," true passion comes from a place of spirit. It's the path of most enjoyment, and if you follow it, you will be living in your passion.

**Rose:** What sort of things bring you joy at the moment?

**Kat:** For me, it's about creating something with other people and watching these things unfold. I need to feel what I'm doing is worthwhile. Right now, I'm co-creating something of service to people in the world. I've always wanted to work more with communities and I'll move towards that in the near future.

## The challenge of co-creating

**Rose:** So living your passion has several different aspects: there's joy and enjoyment; there's co-creating with other people; there's being of service to the world; and then there are ways to work with communities. Do you find co-creating flows easily? I've always found it to be one of the most challenging aspects of soul work, as well one of the most rewarding.

**Kat:** I think everything is co-created. Whether I have a business or I'm working as a team member in a job, I'm still co-creating. It's a really interesting process and people have different styles of co-creating. At one end of the spectrum, there's no plan, no structure at all, just letting it all flow. At the other end, there's a definite plan and structure, goals and timelines. I'm in the middle, where I do like things to flow, but I also need to know we're working together towards some kind of plan. It involves organization, but the organization needs to be free and flexible. It's been very interesting for me to co-create within Positive Elements, because I find when I'm creating something different, or on a higher level, it brings up my "stuff". The co-creative relationship challenges me to look at myself and move through my limitations. I'm used to doing that on my own, but having my project affected by other people's "stuff" is quite new to me, and it has been a challenge. I'm not the most patient person, so I want to it all to happen really fast. Things generally have unfolded quite quickly for me previously, but I've had to learn to be a lot more patient and tolerant with other people, who need to go through some kind of process with issues arising in the business. I've found that a bit tricky.

**Rose:** In order to consciously co-create, it's necessary to do conscious relationship work, work on your own process, remove your own limitations, and look at where you're getting reactive. I've been struck by how many people have said living your passion is fun. My experience is yes, sometimes it is fun, and sometimes it involves looking at our darker side and the places where we get frustrated and maybe feel pain. I don't think you can have growth or learning without occasional discomfort, so I'm glad to hear you saying that's part of it for you.

**Kat:** Definitely! Another thing that comes up for me with co-creating is the commitment. Yes, you have to be passionate about something. Yes, you have to resonate with it, and just do it, but that doesn't mean it's going to be easy. There are times when you come up against blockages, where the process slows and stagnates and "issues" arise. Sometimes I do want to reassess and consider if this is really what I want to be doing. Often, something needs to change internally; I'm approaching it in some way that's not working. I want to take it in this direction, while really it wants to flow that way. Of course there'll be friction, because I'm trying to push it somewhere it's not really going, or I need to change my perception about it. I always find as soon as I become attached to an outcome, for it to be a certain way, that's when I start to get into negative emotion. It always goes better when I let go and say, this is what I'm creating right now but I can't foresee the outcome. I have a vague idea of what it can be, but I'm open for it to be otherwise, if that's best for the project. Yes, definitely, I've learned that this year: to get out of the way and let it all flow through me!

**Rose:** It's quite challenging to keep a balance between flowing with process and having a structure or a plan, isn't it? Knowing when you need to let go, and knowing when you need to focus and push through.

**Kat:** For me, it's about being really present to the feeling right now, because I can feel from an intuitive space what needs to be done. From an egoic space, I may be focused on making this much money or doing things a certain way, rather than asking, what is it I need to be doing right now? I don't always get it right! *Laughter.*

**Rose:** In the process you're developing a lot of skills, tools and understandings.

**Kat:** Yes, that's why I've been doing it!

**Rose:** I think you're in your mid twenties – is that right?

**Kat:** Yes, I'm twenty six.

**Rose:** I'm wondering how you've come so quickly to this place of living your passion and joy?

**Kat:** I guess I've always felt a really strong guiding force in my life, taking me and guiding me in the right direction. It is my choice as well of course. I can choose to go there, or mess around here for a while and go in a few circles. At the same time, I feel I don't have a choice. It just happens. The circumstances of my life change so I'm in that space and exposed to these kinds of people, and involved in those kinds of projects. Coming to New Zealand was a real change for me: both the people I've been exposed to and the experiences. I think the way I met Theresa was synchronicity, and now I'm embarking on a journey with her and other people as well. Being part of the Co-Creators network definitely brought about a real shift in my consciousness in terms of co-creating, so that was quite fundamental too.

**Rose:** When did you come to New Zealand?

**Kat:** I've been here about three years now. My mother decided to emigrate here. I was living in India at the time for about seven months. I always knew I didn't want to go back to England, I never felt it was my home, so I decided to come to New Zealand and visit her for a year and then go on to wherever else. I was planning on going to South America, but I never got there. *Laughter.* I ended up staying here because I knew it was the right place for me.

**Rose:** So you're a traveller?

**Kat:** That's a passion as well. It's not just travelling, it's the different cultures. There's something magical for me about being in so-called developing countries. I guess it's

*Sasha:*
*A Friendliness Seed*

*If I could sow a seed for a WHOLE NEW WORLD it would be a friendliness seed to make a world full of friendliness. Everybody would always have a smile on their face. There'd be plants growing and no one would step on the plants and no one would call each other names. It would always be a sunny place, no one would murder anyone, instead they'd ask politely for what they want. This is really the place to be.*

the rawness of life. It feels real. Whereas, in the West, sometimes it feels we've contrived this whole big complicated situation. In the East, you're going back to simplicity and people being really present and loving and content with what they have. It's always been a real joy to be there amongst those people. I want to go back and live there and spend more time there. It's about getting back to a way of being who we really are.

**Rose:** You knew you weren't getting that in the UK, and there was something missing; something different that you wanted?

**Kat:** Even as a child I thought, what am I doing here? I felt very alienated, always feeling, "this is a crazy place, I don't want to be here." Now looking back, I think I had a bit of a negative impression and it's not necessarily like that. I'm sure it's possible to have beautiful experiences there, but I think, generally there is a lack of consciousness; a dark, heavy energy, and a lot of self destructive behavior; people sabotaging themselves with drugs and alcohol. At least that's what I didn't like about it. Then coming to New Zealand, there's just that lightness of being! It's not always totally so, I mean there are problems here too, but there's so much more space in which to expand your awareness!

**Rose**: So tell me a bit about Positive Elements.

**Kat:** I got involved just over a year ago now. I met Theresa when we went on a trip down the Wanganui River together, an incredible journey, which transformed a lot of my life at the time. The river has a really strong energy and it created a shift, a realigning in me. It was a beautiful, quite intense couple of days. When I came back everything turned itself on its head. My flat felt all wrong and I had to move out of Auckland to the countryside, to the Waitakere Ranges. I left my job and all my security. *Laughter*

**Rose:** A big leap?

**Kat:** Yes, a leap of faith. I guess I'm getting better at doing that because I watch how, if you take that first step into the unknown, the Universe just picks you up and runs with you. Suddenly all this magic happens in your life! It's about trusting! I started doing some bits and pieces for

Theresa because she needed help, and I got more and more involved with Positive Elements as time went on. It felt like a vision that's been in my heart for quite a long time. Sometimes I feel it's my reason for being here on the planet, or one of the reasons. In the biggest sense it's about human potential and supporting the unfolding of this potential. It's also about creating wealth and opportunities for everybody involved, from the communities we work with, to the people who are part of the business. Whoever comes into contact with that organization gains wealth and opportunity, maybe in a financial sense, and also in terms of learning, growth, and development. More specifically, the business side of things is sustainable products that are handmade by village co-operatives. We promote them in New Zealand and Australia and now internationally as well. That's the economic wheel.

**Rose:** These are village co-operatives in places like India?

**Kat:** At the moment, we're only working in India, but we've set ourselves a big task, working with communities and businesses all over the world. It's quite a big dream! Why not aim high and go for it! *Laughter.* And it's happening, so it's really exciting!

It's about creating opportunities and wealth for the communities, providing them with a livelihood that's rewarding and develops their skills, because it's quite hard for them to survive sometimes. Further down the track my interest lies in a percentage of the profits going into a foundation, which will give back to those communities we're working with. It could be in a financial way, but more so, in services provided. For example, there might be a fund for starting enterprises in a new community, so they can afford equipment or training. But more than that, my vision is for all these little communities all over the world, to be able to network and come together with all the people who are buying the products, to create this one big global network, as a forum for transformation and learning.

## An exchange of learning

**Rose:** It's about connecting communities and supporting people in the Third World to become more economically sustainable?

**Kat:** There's been a lot of talk about sustainability and sustainable business in the last few years. The subject of sustainability is such a huge complicated issue; everyone has different interpretations of it. Some say sustainability is about living off your backyard and not using a car, while other people think sustainability is about people's development and growth. There's so much in it, we feel we don't want to be putting our focus there so much anymore. The people in these communities have an amazing amount of joy and inner contentment. They know what it's like to be in community. They live a lot in the moment, being present and having fun, and that's what we can learn from them. So I guess it's really about providing an environment for an exchange of learning. Rather than we Westerners helping people, it's more about helping each other and growing together.

**Rose:** You also have a big, wonderful global vision, connecting people around the planet. Have you actually met the people in the Indian communities?

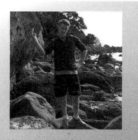

*Ben: A Talent Seed*

*If I would plant a seed for a whole new world I would plant a talent seed. Every being has a talent seed to plant. It would grow into a world of people with countless talents and ideas to express and share with many great friends.*

**Kat:** I haven't been to Auroville yet, where our products are made, but I have lived in similar communities in India and Africa, as a volunteer, and I always found I got far more back from the service than I ever put in. You get back so much joy and learning. You realize it's not about helping them; it's about helping yourself and them! That's what we'd like to convey through Positive Elements. It's about what we can all learn.

**Rose:** What's happening with Positive Elements at the moment?

**Kat:** A lot of business development! Right now we're taking on investors and creating the company. That's one thread. Another is marketing: how do we get our story across? How do we engage people? We're developing the systems, the team and the operations. It's pretty huge! *Laughter.* It's been an amazing experience. I've learned so much I know I'll be using in the future, because I don't see this being my only project. Once this is set up and running, I can take a backseat. I'm still going to be involved in it because it's very dear to my heart, but there are lots of other projects and business ideas I'm interested in too. It's been a great experience to find out what's involved in starting a business and how you develop one and get it to a point where it's successful. Learning how to do that in a different, more conscious way and from the heart, that's new learning for all of us!

**Rose:** It is! You sound like a woman with a mission!

**Kat:** Yes! I think that's my journey in life. I know I'm here to create things. I know everybody's path is different and mine's not better than others, but I do feel mine is an active journey. I can flip into manic doing, because I've always been a very driven person, wanting to achieve a lot in my life. Now I'm asking why? Why am I trying to achieve this? Am I trying to get some sort of approval? I've come to the realization it's really not about what you achieve in this life; it's the process of doing it. Am I enjoying this process? Am I really learning from this process of creating a business? I'm trying to stay in that place of being, while doing. I do struggle with it!

## Fostering joy

**Rose:** You've said joy is an important part of it for you. What have you learned about what fosters joy or what prevents it?

**Kat:** Joy is about being present. Being really present in whatever I do. I lose joy when I'm striving, and then the process becomes heavy and doesn't flow. It's about really appreciating life, appreciating every moment, and realizing what an amazing opportunity it is to be part of this! Yes, it's not always easy, and there are challenges, but I'm surrounded by all these incredibly inspiring people. I guess I feel the joy when I lose the expectations. When I lose the expectations, and I'm really real with what is right now, how beautiful it is and how lucky I am! It's a deeper experience of life.

**Rose:** Remembering and being grateful; so we don't lose sight of how wonderful everything is.

**Kat:** It's also about being in connection. I need to stay aware of doing things that nurture me, like meditation, walking, or having time to myself. Without those things I can't experience joy. If I'm not connected spiritually, joy isn't quite there. It's a more fickle emotion; happiness if something goes right, disappointment if it goes wrong; rather than feeling the joy of living.

**Rose:** Do you have a spiritual practice that supports you to be present?

**Kat**: I do meditation but I don't think it has to be just about a strict spiritual practice. What's spiritual for me is being in nature or dancing, or any of those things that uplift me. Meditation is very important to me, although I don't always do it! I know meditating makes me feel so amazing and enables me to give so much more of myself in the world, but I still wake up in the morning thinking, ah no, I don't feel like doing it! It's a challenge to make the effort sometimes. It has to be a routine; wake up and just do it, because as soon as you get out of the routine, it's so much harder to get back into it.

**Rose:** It all comes back to maintaining personal consciousness!

**Kat:** If I get back to the roots of why we're actually here, it doesn't matter what I do in my life, what I create, whether I create a vision or not, but did I become more conscious in the process?

**Rose**: Yes! The central purpose is to become more conscious and we all have our own particular ways of doing that. For some, it's about community; for others, it's developing businesses or writing books, or whatever. Do you have a big dream for your personal future?

**Kat:** I get a feeling of it; it's already real to me on some level. It's a feeling is of living a really incredible life. There's abundance, money is no longer an issue. I can live the life I want to live, travelling a lot, being in communities, setting up things in different countries. I also see, in the future, I'll be playing more of a public role as well, more out there, speaking in public, in the media, at conferences; things like that. Putting myself out there, in the public eye, is the one thing that brings up some fear in me but it's something I'm starting to explore now, learning to be comfortable with who I am and express myself to larger groups of people. I feel it's going to be an incredible life, full of magic and wonderful people.

The way I see it is, we can choose whatever reality we want in this life. Why not choose the most amazing? It's all about how high we set your sights, really. We often limit ourselves far too much in what we think we can achieve. Sometimes it's unconscious. For instance, over this lifetime, I've had issues with money. Money to me hasn't been something good. I thought having money was selfish. All this stuff! So I was limiting myself to a life of not having money because I had negative associations with it. I've been working on turning that around because actually there's nothing wrong with money at all! It's just energy. Now I feel really comfortable saying, well yes, I do want to have money. But it's not just about money; it's about being able to live an extraordinary life. I aspire to stay in places that are amazing, to go to places that are amazing, and to be surrounded by amazing things and people. It's a whole way of being.

**Rose:** Do you feel positive about the future of the planet as well as your own personal future?

**Kat:** I'm very, very optimistic about the future of the planet. I envision a whole new way of being together in the world, in harmony. I'm really excited about the changes I see happening, and I see so much happening! People are doing such incredible things in the world. Everyone is contributing in their own way, whether it's big or small. I feel there's a whole shift in consciousness happening, and we can choose the reality we want to live in. If you want to live in a world that's utopian, you will move in that direction and surround yourself with those kinds of people. Right now I'm sitting here on Waiheke Island, which is close to paradise on Earth! That's what I've chosen to have as my reality. Other people live in a different reality and think the future is something to be feared, and it's all going to get worse with massive chaos, death and destruction. And, of course, that's happening in the world. I imagine places like Iraq and Palestine must be hell on Earth. It seems the planet is kind of splitting into two dimensions. On one side, there's the dark reality, and on the other, there's the light reality; and they're both happening at exactly the same time. Do you want to be in the reality of love, or do you want to be in the reality of fear? You just need to choose which one you're in!

**Rose:** You've made some good choices, Kat!

## *We're responsible for our own energy*

**Kat**: I try not to expose myself to things that bring up fear, because I know I can go there if I pick up a paper or watch the news. We are responsible for our own energy and I want to keep my energy as high as possible. To be able to function in that high energy I need to be in an environment that supports me. I feel very blessed to be surrounded by a group of people who are always reminding me of who I really am, of the best person I can be; because I forget. That's what I think co-creation is about: supporting each other in our process of unfolding. And reminding each other; bringing each other back into love, back into thinking of ourselves as divine, supporting each other in our transformation.

> *Original source of creation, the void of all that is*
> *Thank you for the breath of life*
> *Thank you for my gifts*
> *Sacred mystery, touch my heart*
> *In beauty may I walk*
> *Great mystery, be my guide*
> *So that I may walk my talk*
> *Original source remain with me*
> *So that I may always feel the warmth*
> *Of your eternal flame*
> *Deep within my soul.*
> Sacred Path Tarot Cards - created by Jamie Sams

**Baba Nam Kevalam, Love is all there is.**

### *We are being called to become One Global Family*

Only a transformation of consciousness will ensure our survival as a species and an adequate quality of life for future generations. It's a shift from "me" and "mine" to "all of us are in this together."

All over the world, people are waking up to the need to discover and create new ways of co-existence on Planet Earth. We recognize the problems faced by humanity are shared, and solutions will only be found by moving towards new ways of experiencing ourselves as One Global Family.

# Shift Three

## From feeling trapped by circumstances to the recognition life is a journey of courage, trust, and discovery, and we are creators capable of making conscious choices.

When we hear the call of the inner life, and set out on our journey to find life's meaning and purpose, we learn to travel in deeper and more radical trust, shedding old psychological skins and our need to be in control. As we become simpler, we experience at a deeper level our essential loving nature and the interconnectedness of everything. We realize there are myriad possibilities latent in each moment, and peace of mind and fulfillment rest, not so much in having what we want, as in consciously choosing to be aligned with authentic values.

# David Dwyer
## Hello world!

At an early age David experienced a deep connection and communion with nature. This led him to a profound crisis of values about humanity's destruction of nature, and a conflict between his moral conscience and the education he was offered. As a consequence, he left school at sixteen and took to the road on a journey of adventure and discovery. He is a passionate community gardener, a vegetarian and vegan cook, and a performance artist. He has a vision for establishing permaculture in Golden Bay.

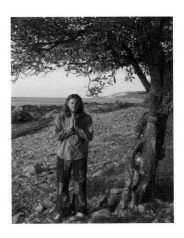

Before my conversation with David, I was fascinated to know how a conscious twenty-two year old, setting out on the journey into adulthood, makes sense of the conflicts and contradictions of our 21st century world. Some twenty year olds these days are very much more conscious and emotionally mature than earlier generations at a similar age. Yet in New Zealand, the suicide rate amongst young men is one of the highest in the world. This surely suggests there is some way in which families and the education system are not meeting the needs of the young.

**David:** Living my passion means being able to take my spiritual ideals and put them into something tangible. The whole concept of permaculture has introduced me to that possibility. I believe in not harming anything, living in harmony with the natural world and nurturing the environment. I really believe we're born with everything available and we can choose what we do with that. If it means covering the earth with concrete, then what we get is a whole lot of concrete, but if we want to look at the beauty of what's already there and live in harmony with it, then we can live on a diverse Earth full of life.

Recently I've been having really strong messages to go to Takaka, Takaka, Takaka! I went there about five years ago when I was seventeen, for a Rainbow Gathering, and had an absolutely amazing time. I've never been back since then and I certainly hadn't anticipated going to live there any time soon. But I'm getting this calling to go and live there for some years to establish permaculture. I've looked up Takaka in Wikipedia and it said it's the home of alternative culture, vegan and vegetarian cafes and organic farms.

Since I made the decision to go I've discovered many friends are having a similar calling at the moment. I started getting emails from people I hadn't heard from in a long time talking about the rich dark soil in Golden Bay! So you can expect a lot of young, enthusiastic, nature loving people to be in Golden Bay in the future, and we're going with a vision of permaculture. I think it's a really suitable place. Whenever I think about it, I get very excited. Something's telling me, go for it!

**Rose:** Do you think the most important thing you can do is to work with the earth?

**David:** Yes, and at the same time, I recognize there's a sense of personal inner evolution, or inner self knowing, self realization I guess, that's not dependent on any outer activity. It doesn't matter what I'm doing in the world necessarily. I feel at peace when I'm in touch with my true self, and just by doing that, I'm sharing myself with the whole Universe and constantly becoming more blissful.

But I am on the Earth and I feel really glad to be here and to have the opportunity to share. I guess to be honest, I've found since I was pretty young, I've really struggled to fit into societal habits and have felt quite bitter at times that I felt somewhat obligated to be part of the destruction of the Earth by living in the normal way. To discover ways I can have a lifestyle which doesn't involve destroying the Earth, which I love, is a reason to live, really. I thought through all the logical conclusions when I was a young teenager and decided the best thing I could do to respect the Earth and all life that I loved, would be to end my life. I couldn't see any way of not living the way society lives and destroying what I love, so there seemed no point in living. I had to really look at that dilemma and I grew out of it mainly through meeting other people who had similar feelings and thoughts. Then I realized, oh, ok, I'm not totally alone and there is something I can do which is positive. So this move to Takaka is something positive I can do and it's tangible!

**Rose:** Sounds like as a teenager you didn't want to be part of a destructive world and didn't know how you could be true to yourself within that. Part of you wanted to die, but you made a conscious decision no, you could actually live and do something positive. Were these difficult times for you, David?.

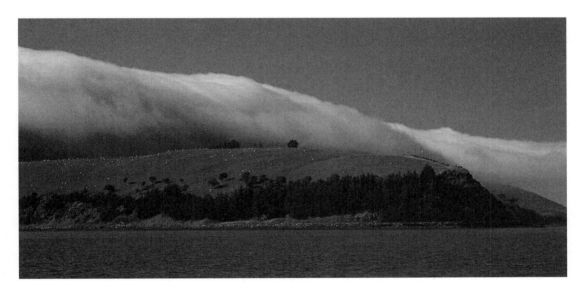

**David:** I was asked to leave school because I was considered a bad influence. I was living in my own world in which schoolwork was not a priority and enticing people to join me. Connecting with nature was my priority, as was being a kind but free and creative individual. There were certain teachers in the school I really connected with who inspired me. Then there were many others who had a more authoritarian approach and there was no healthy way of relating with them, really.

**Rose:** They asked you to leave school because you were a kind, nature-loving person?

**David:** Well, perhaps because my individuality was uncompromising.

**Rose:** Did you speak up for yourself a lot?

**David:** I don't think it was so much that but, for example, on a mufti day when we could wear whatever we wanted, I wore a girl's kilt to school as my mufti and a jester's hat, some friends of mine were doing a band performance and I got up to dance. I was a bit of an exhibitionist, not because I wanted to show anything, just because I wanted to be free and I saw no reason not to be. I guess I was possibly a bit too 'full-on', or maybe a bit intimidating, I'm not sure. Also, I was open about a desire to go and live with the apes in South America, thinking perhaps a complete immersion in nature may be the only way to escape the deep pangs of my conscience. This desire came from a deep dissatisfaction with human culture. I still remember Ms Garden's response after she had asked me what I wanted to do when I left school: "Well, we really can't help you then!" To be perfectly honest, I think the principal of that school and the teachers could tell I had no interest in schoolwork. They could see there was no reason for me to be there. I thoroughly wanted to leave and the only reason I was staying at that point was because my parents wanted me to, and I didn't realize I had another option. So when I was asked to leave my response was: "Really! Hello world!"

**Rose:** It troubles me the school system couldn't tolerate you being different.

**David:** Also, they weren't providing an environment stimulating enough for me. I would happily spend my days walking in the bush and learn a lot more than I would at school. I could really feel from the earth. When I hit puberty, and started to really come into the world, look around me and think a lot, I discovered there's a natural presence in nature. When I was walking in the bush, I was constantly in awe just looking at the trees, or I'd stop and look at a bug for five or ten minutes. I felt I was being invited into the world by the earth, and it was not rushing me, was not pressuring me to do anything, just showing me how to be, and teaching me all the most important lessons about myself, about how to live in harmony. In a really natural way I felt I was being shown into a richer life. The time I spent in school was just the opposite; all this information and the message that you're nothing unless you know this. I was looking around at what society was doing, and the school seemed essentially to be working towards the destruction of the Earth by training more workers for the industries that are destroying everything. So I was thinking, why in hell would I want to be part of that? There's no reason for me to want to have anything to do with this whatsoever! I wrote poetry and sat in corners on my own, and I wasn't the only person doing that.

**Rose:** Did you feel isolated, lonely?

**David:** Well, at the original high school I went to, I didn't find it hard to make friends, but I felt very alone when it came to what was important to me. Then I met some other people who went to a different school, who were questioning more and were much more environmentally minded. They didn't work so much or get into rugby and alcohol; they were more theatrical people who liked to improvise theatre sports. They were far more creative, expressive, and liberally minded people, and I liked them so much and formed such strong friendships with them, I changed schools against the wishes of my parents. That's where I was eventually asked to leave, because I was too different for the alternative school!

**Rose:** So amongst your peers, there were a lot of people simply conforming?

**David:** Yes, it was a social enslavement. I shifted schools a lot because my family was moving. We moved from Australia to New Zealand, and then I went to three new schools in four or five years in Dunedin and Christchurch. It meant I never got tied into the social side of it, because I was always a new person coming into a brand new social scene, so I could easily see how unique I was. Everyone is unique, but sometimes if you're in one school you can get a little more indoctrinated by the social structure and find some comfort in that. There was no comfort for me because I was always coming into an awkward, brand new environment. I learned to deal with that, which in the long run was really healthy, because I developed some skills which everyone eventually learns when they go out into the world. Some people stay with their comfortable group of friends after they leave school. Personally, I think that's quite sad.

**Rose:** I'm struck by how you felt really at home with nature, with the earth, but alienated from society, from people. You left school at sixteen?

**David:** Yes, there was a brief moment, pretty much the only time I've been depressed, right after I left school. I had no idea what I was going to do and my parents just didn't "get it." I found out later they were having their own problems. They were very private in their lives so I guess I didn't find myself opening up to them. Yet, at the same time I was really blatant, I didn't hide anything from them either. I became vegetarian at fourteen and vegan at fifteen or sixteen. There was a brief moment of depression when I was drinking my father's home-brew and I had a shed where I used to record music with microphones all over the wall. My parents said, "Get a job and start doing something to become part of ordinary worldly activity, or else go!" So I thought, "Ok, I'll go then," and I hit the road hitchhiking. I had a really deep sense, which I recognized as my heart's intuition, and I've become more familiar with now, I had a sense everything was ok. It was all happening the way it was, as it needed to, and I would go on a journey, and I would discover things. It was just time to go on a journey.

**Rose:** Brave of you!

**David:** It was quite brave, but I didn't have any fear, so I didn't really feel I needed to be brave. It was a lot more exciting and less painful than being caught up in watching the world being destroyed and not knowing what to do about it.

**Rose:** Did you follow your intuition on the journey?

**David:** Yeah, it was amazing! There were people out in the world I didn't know existed who were thinking about all sorts of things: parts of the Bible that had been lost, conspiracy theories, all this stuff for me to engage my mind with and think, "Ah what! This isn't how they told me it is!" I could hardly take it all in!

**Rose:** Sounds like a true education.

**David:** It was an incredible education! I hitched all around the South Island for the next few years; that's how I discovered the Rainbow Gathering in Takaka. For the summer, I'd go out and around the north part of the South Island. In winter I'd go down to Dunedin and stay with friends and busk. I started playing a little shaman drum a friend had given me, and I'd bang on it and sing songs about whatever was inside me and what I believed in, make a bit of money and get a bag of peanuts, or whatever. That was the beginning of my performance career! The most inspiring thing was when I went hitchhiking with no money and I discovered if I believed I would be provided with everything I needed, I was! Every time! All the time! A huge part of that was realizing how little I needed. I would get so much freedom in my mind, and my whole being, from not having this constant river of desires flowing into me. I must have this, and this, and now I need a coffee. I must have a big dinner every day, and I need to be stimulated by the Internet or watching tv. Having nothing gave me this amazing freedom! Not having money is so inspiring for the mind! You don't even think about money, you have no relationship with it, whatsoever! It's astounding what a huge part of your mind money takes up! Without it, you're just free, never knowing what you're going to do next! Having no idea what you're going to do tomorrow or even in an hour! That's how free you are! Everything becomes open. It's inspiring beyond anything!

Another thing is physically being in the open air, being able to look around you any time, free from the four walls of a house, looking around and seeing a 360 degree vision of sky. You just feel wild! I lay down under trees with only an old sleeping bag for warmth. When I'd stand on the side of the road hitchhiking, sometimes it would be quite cold, especially as I had bare feet, so I learned how to relax, and if I could relax I wouldn't be so cold. If I started getting really cold, I could just shake my whole body and dance hard out at the side of the road and warm up in no time. Simple things like that make me feel safe. The thought, if I don't have a jersey I'll freeze, is completely imaginary.

**Rose:** You learned to be very self reliant and not need very much at all?

**David:** Anything I did need came to me. I didn't ask for food. People just gave, and if not I'd live off fruit trees, nut trees, and other edible stuff I'd find. I did a bit of seasonal fruit picking work for a few weeks.

**Rose:** Did you ever feel scared?

**David:** Yes, there were a couple of times when I found it hard. I guess we all fear the unknown. Sometimes, when I thought I needed to make a decision, I'd get a bit perplexed and not know what to do, but there've been very few times when I was afraid; very, very few. I know now the only thing to fear is fear itself. I get a great sense of fearlessness and freedom from knowing if somebody was to attack me and take my physical life on the street, or whatever, the only thing to make that a really horrible experience would be fear of losing my life. I'm just not going to be afraid of that; there's no real suffering in it.

**Rose:** Your whole experience of journeying has been wonderful in itself; at the same time do you feel it's preparing you for something?

**David:** Absolutely. When I was growing up, we had a Christian orientation but very unorthodox, quite beautiful and natural. It showed me a real love of God. I don't resonate to be part of the formal structure of the church, but I recognize what's happening in each heart, and I recognize my family is the whole of humanity. Travelling has shown me I can find my equality with anyone, and I love to do that. Just living has been a preparation in that sense. Also if the world does take on drastic changes, which it may, and is doing, I feel I'm getting better and better at living in a way which is an example of living without compromise. I intend to participate in the healing of the Earth, so we can look to living here for a longer period of time. Also, there's a real inner preparation of learning to know myself in my eternal nature and remembering who I am.

**Rose:** How do you feel about the times we live in? Are you optimistic?

**David:** Oh absolutely! I'm completely optimistic. I believe there is divine justice in everything. To the question why the Earth is being destroyed by humans, I've looked at it, and realized many people living today weren't the creators of this. It's been something which has been put in motion by our ancestors, and I say it's waiting for enough people to realize real true self knowledge so we don't need to go driving everywhere, rushing around like rats to get material wealth. We're discovering something much deeper and more fulfilling. I think it's a real evolutionary process. We're being given choices all the time. Humanity can't choose to be peaceful without having the other option available as well.

**Rose:** It has to be a real choice.

**David:** Yes, it's a real choice and I think that's healthy. I love everybody. Discovering that hasn't been a choice, it's been a discovery, and it's given me a great sense of peace. Sometimes people gather socially and they're thinking, these people are a little bit better than those other people, and they always find something a little bit dissatisfying when they make criticisms. I say, "oh, but I like them because of this", and they go, "you love everyone!" and I say, "I do! Being part of my social club means not excluding anyone. Sorry, this isn't a private club!"

**Rose:** This alone will create a very beautiful, satisfying and fulfilling life for you.

## Post-script

A few weeks after the interview, David sent me the following thoughts. I find what he has to say so moving and so important I am adding it here.

**David:** The words you wrote before the interview touched very close to my heart; almost like something I would have intended to write in a book someday, but which obviously needs to be heard now. New Zealand has such a high suicide rate for young people, particularly men. I have looked at some of the statistics and from what I gather men accomplish attempted suicides far more than women in New Zealand, and no doubt worldwide. Maybe men are more likely than women to have the physical means to suicide. Or, are women more open to the support that may flood their way in the case of an attempted suicide or at the hint it may be on their mind? Perhaps women are more communicative about their struggles in general, giving more opportunity for support?.

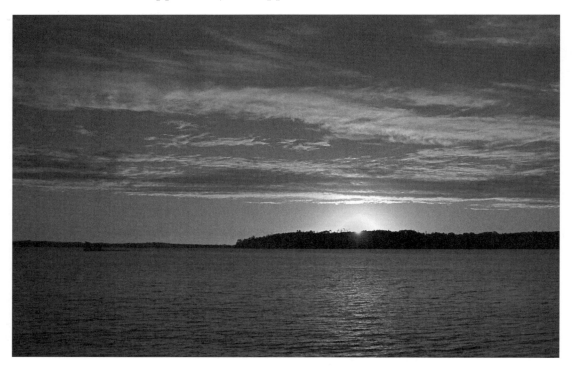

I understood my life within modern societal patterns would be destructive of "life" (living things) and hence recognized logically to continue my personal life as it was would destroy life (living things). This, for me, was merely the catalyst to make a choice not to live in a way which disagreed with my conscience, and instead to live in alignment with my own personal moral understandings, even if they were not in alignment with the actions of those around me. I did not ever have an actual desire to die. Although I had made a logical conclusion of the moral value of me doing so, it would have taken an emotional commitment. Frankly, I love living things too much. It was only a matter of time before I remembered I am a living thing too and that the separation between humanity and nature is purely imaginary. I had not even the slightest notion I could live a life that would nurture nature and benefit the Earth! I never once glimpsed any opportunity throughout my schooling for positive interaction with nature, in fact had I done so my attitude would have been transformed. The schools seemed to me uninterested in real planet Earth. Had I any glimmer of hope the school I was attending could actually help me live a life in alignment with my moral conscience, I would have seized it with both hands and paid absolute attention. My values had nothing to do with money or survival on a small scale, they were about survival on a big scale, survival for the future of everything with responsible actions in the short term. Our school system is still based on the old Victorian style of education. Is it because old habits die hard? Because we fear the unknown?

Turning that overwhelming frustration into a passion for positive action has been a huge part of my journey, and an incredibly trans-formative process. Ultimately it has led me to an acceptance of everything (nearly) that bothers me about humanity. Self responsibility has presented me with the greatest challenge. We are creative beings; in that we have no choice. Choosing to create positively with harmless intent is possibly the most important responsibility we have as individuals and as a whole.

Children are the light of this world. In fact they are the light of heaven for the world to see. Children are so perfectly frank and open, they have an abrupt honesty that cuts away the dross and makes simple things bright and wonderful.

I have commented on the actions of society on a material plane that, as a youth, disturbed me so much I removed myself from having an "ordinary life". Since then, I have come to recognize the spirit in which we live is of the utmost importance, not the materials we alter. However if we accept that spiritual powers will save the world, which they will, surely we can see that one who is in full appreciation of spirit's perfect bliss has no desire to offer their physical self anything that is not simple and pure.

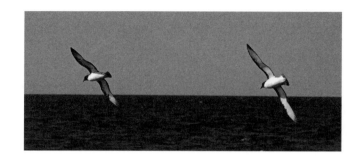

*People are in essence beautiful*
*Those that hide their beauty*
*Hide their essence*
*Those that do not see beauty*
*Do not see much.*

Love, David

# We each make a difference

*The transformation of consciousness*
*begins inside each one of us.*

*Our states of mind, emotional energy, and daily actions*
*affect the wholes of which we are a part.*

*The larger whole may be a relationship,*
*family, work team, nation, or the entire world.*

*Whether our thoughts and actions*
*are positive, negative,*
*or apathetic, they all factor in.*

*We can choose to make a difference by making*
*a commitment to living more consciously.*

*This means living nonviolently, becoming aware*
*of our limited and judgmental thinking*
*and emotional reactivity,*
*healing ourselves and redeeming our lost powers.*

# *Shift Four*

## Withdrawing energy from what is not working and instead putting attention on what we choose to create.

Focusing primarily on what is not working in the world, or in our lives, leads to cycles of reactivity and disempowerment. When we choose to use our dissatisfactions to fuel our passion for positive change and focus wholeheartedly on what we choose to create, in alignment with higher values, we become pro-active and maximally empowered.

# *Will Lau*
## Punching through the fear

Born in a little village on the far side of Hong Kong, Will lived most of his early life in sunny Napier, a coastal town in Hawkes Bay, New Zealand, where he moved at age three. Educated in Canterbury University with an Honours degree in Mechanical Engineering, he embarked on a career as a healthcare product designer before taking an unexpected detour down the road of entrepreneurship, after a backpacking adventure that transformed his life. In a five year whirlwind he competed in an international technology space, to found three start-ups, the latest of which, he led 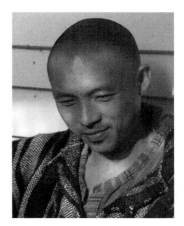 to seven figure profitability within three years, before taking another detour. Will is presently on a nomadic journey of adventure which encompasses his loves of technology, entrepreneurship and his own spiritual self discovery.

**Will:** Living my passion is about having the courage to do what I really want to do in life. Passion for me isn't a fire from within, it's this massive energy that consumes me and I don't have a choice. After university, I did a career path: five years of learning mechanical engineering. I then went on to what was a pretty good job as a product designer for Fisher and Paykel Healthcare division. It was interesting to me, but it wasn't fully living my passion. I went overseas and did some re-thinking and when I came back, it all came to a crunch point. To make the jump from what other people, and myself actually, expected me to do, to doing what I really wanted to do, was a big decision, probably the hardest of my life.

**Rose:** When you say it was a crunch point, what happened? How did you get to the crunch?

**Will:** I came back realizing I had a passion for technology and a specific kind of technology, PDAs (Personal Digital Assistants), which were about to take over the whole world at the time. When I was travelling and backpacking, I took one of these PDAs and started conversations with people in the industry. When I got back, I really wanted to get into the industry so I started pumping up, getting the cash flow going with my old job to give the bank balance some life support. Meanwhile at night, I learned to programme, not because programming interested me in itself, but because I loved the industry, and I wanted to learn everything about it. Ultimately, one of the guys I connected with in the technology world asked me if I could revamp the website for his start-up. I didn't know how to create websites at the time, but my best friend was a graphic designer, so I thought, ok, I can subcontract it all out to people I know, but at least I can coordinate everything and I'll be doing something in this industry. That was my start. After that I got referrals for my work.

At night, I was working forty hours a week on websites and in the day I was working forty hours a week at my job. It wasn't too bad, because my nighttime forty hours was like my playtime! It was easy to see where my energy was strongest.

Ultimately, a time came when two major contracts came in and I wanted to pitch for both of them. If I won either contract, I would not have enough time to deliver on the contract and do my day job. As there was a one month notice on my job, I essentially needed to quit my job, hang it all on the line, and hope I would win one of those contracts to keep me fed!

I went through the point of thinking; I'm essentially throwing away the entire ten years of my career path! My bank balance wasn't so great at the time and I had a very large mortgage, so my mind was saying, "If I pitch at these contracts, they'll pay ok, but then I don't know where my next dollar will be coming from!" Ultimately, I just had to do it, because I'd lost interest in my job.

That was the crunch and I made the decision to follow my passion. You know, it took eighteen months to get over the sheer joy of not being in the nine-to-five, that'd hit me each morning. The joy of playing each day has not ended. You read books which say passion is like playing and it is like that!

**Rose**: What is it about technology you find so fascinating?

**Will**: Well, technology is fast moving. It's always changing. It matches my patience. I don't really have a lot of attention and patience for a project that doesn't move and shift and change a lot. Technology changes every day. I often start my day for an hour or so reading in Technology News about all the latest developments. It's a different world and, back then when I was a little younger, the world of technology held huge glamour for me. I'm talking about this bigger picture of the start-up, where you're forging new ground, pioneering stuff. In this space, you're giving it your all, totally living in it. Then there's the story of rags to riches, like Hollywood in a way. You make it big. You're a name on the map. On top of that, technology is fascinating to me. There's so much learning. So, there's all the glamour, and I also get off on the technology. Some people are attracted to shiny jewels and beads; I'm attracted to things with buttons! It's in my nature.

**Rose**: It sounds very dynamic, always stretching you.

**Will:** Yes, it is. It's always different every day.

**Rose**: When did you make your leap of trust?

**Will:** February 2000, one year to the day since I'd left to go backpacking, I created a web design company with myself being the sole employee, and in came the contracts.

**Rose**: Did you get both contracts you were pitching for?

**Will:** Yes, I won both contracts and they paid the equivalent of half a year's salary for me. That's when I realized living your passion is about courage. I scanned back over the year and looked at the profound shift in the way I was

*Louisa: A New World Kindness Seed*

*If I can sow a seed for a new world it would be a seed of kindness. The world that will come out of this loyal seed would be full of kindness with no murder and no stealing. People would work hard for the money they earn. They would volunteer to help rebuild and repaint old houses. Everyone would do a good part for this wonderful world. When anyone gets hurt, someone would come and help them. If anyone is deeply sick but cannot afford the payment, the hospital would do a fundraiser for the family, and of course families would show true kindness and donate money for the sick person. If it's still not enough, the hospital would take the amount raised and help cure the sickness for this person anyway.*

living, and it all boiled down to courage. When I went backpacking, I wasn't like the average Kiwi who can't wait to go. It was more, "oh well, I suppose I should go. I don't want to be here thirty years down the track not even having seen the world." It was more a "to do", pushing myself out of my comfort zone and facing some of my fears. I came back buzzing, realizing how amazing it is to travel, and how amazing it was to face those fears, so they had no hold on me. Then I started getting into this thing I do when there's a decision to be made, or I'm sensing a bit of fear, when I'm weighing up between left or right, one direction or another, I'll go in the direction where there's most fear, because I know that will bring new experiences and learning.

## The Warrior's way

**Rose:** What have you discovered from doing that?

**Will:** You expand your comfort, and in terms of your passion, you break through all the barriers holding you back. Those initial barriers are generally financial, "I don't want to do this, because I'll have to give up my job and my financial security." Then all these excuses come up. I've seen it in so many people.

**Rose**: So living your passion has been a personal growth journey for you, and at least part of what motivates you is to move through your fears and barriers?

**Will:** Oh yes, totally! It's the warrior's paradigm. I use a kind of warrior energy to punch through, but there's a lot of play involved as well.

**Rose**: You had a radical first shift when you left your career path and set up your own business. Didn't you have a second shift recently, when you became involved with the Co-Creators network?

**Will**: Yes, that's another example of punching through the fear. I had a space of two years, when I absolutely loved every moment. I was learning so much and travelling around the world with my laptop in my backpack. I was contracted to American companies and earning money I never thought I could earn so easily. Then I had a second phase of going into bigger businesses, and ultimately one caught me into one spot and anchored me down so I couldn't leave. It was a business partnership that became quite unhealthy. I was burnt out from the relationship and the passion started leaving me. When the passion left, it became work. When you're working eighty hours a week and you're not having fun, you burn out. So things came to a crunch for the second time and I walked out. I didn't sell my share of the company, but I exited day-to-day operations fully. It's quite a scary thing to be in a space with nothing to go to: going into the empty. I'd left my life in Auckland, all my friends, all the people and relationships I'd built up over the previous seven or eight years. My partner at the time, had an alternative outlook on life, which was quite scary and alien to me, but over time I started feeling at home in that more spiritual space.

**Rose:** Is this when spirituality first became important for you? Has it emerged as you've made these life changing shifts?

**Will:** I feel it was there before; however my own authentic walk has been more recent. Mum was a born-again Christian, so I had a real taste of that in my teens. But it wasn't right for me. In my partner, I was very much seeing the same patterns of how spirit works, that played in my mum's life. I was revisiting in a different flavor and style and I realized there are many different styles of spiritual path. Later, when my partner and I had broken up for a while, I read "*The Celestine Prophecy.*" When I finished it, I thought "Gee! I wonder if this is true. Alright then let's test it! Ok, Universe, if this is true; I want the insights in this book to start playing out in my life, starting now!" Almost immediately my life became an amazing ride of one synchronicity after another. It was very exciting! The next thing I knew, I was on this big journey of discovery! I journeyed everywhere, circled the country three times that year, and over to Australia. I took off for a year and a half, and I guess I'm still journeying now!

**Rose**: When you've taken these leaps, what have you found inside yourself that has enabled that courage?

**Will:** It's that warrior thing. Scary yes, but hey! Let's do it anyway! It's actually the passion energy, the fire. For me passion is a flame. The most passionate people tend to be really fiery. They take the flame, direct it at what they're scared of, and just blow right through it. The fear holds no power under the flame. I've also seen other people use a different way. My ex-partner does it through surrendering into a deep place, until she hits the bottom. Again, in that surrender, you realize the fear holds no power. For me, it's the fire. That's what gets me through. Using the flame and surrendering are decisions to face and defeat our fear, and when we do that, we find ourselves "in the empty." That's quite a hard place to be and you can be there for a while. It's like jumping off a cliff; once you've jumped you can't change your mind and try to fly out. It's too late, you've done it! At that point, you just have to hold your fire and contain it.

## Creating the new culture

**Rose:** Yes, I recognize the process of surrender, "being in the empty", and having to contain the creative fire. Putting language to these experiences is all part of learning about the creative process so we can work with it more consciously. Going back to your passion for technology, would you say computers are good tools for creating a new culture and a peaceful future?

**Will:** It's already happened! The new culture's been created and has been running for seven years now, since the first dot.com boom. People don't see this because they're not deeply involved in it. For example, I went on a cruise we won through one of our retailers and I bumped into a guy from New Zealand. He and his wife were living in the States and had a company of twenty people. He'd met his business partner who is American in the 90's through Newsgroups, a place on the Internet where you can post things onto a bulletin board and people can reply and have discussions. They started emailing each other, working on software and projects. Then they started creating a project together and ultimately he flew to the States to check it out and loved it. The next thing you know, a few years later they had this company.

Another example, I had a business in which I never met my business partner. He was Croatian. I emailed him and talked to him on the phone. We created the most anticipated product of 2001 in our industry, which paid off half my mortgage. Those kinds of relationships play a part in how businesses start. We hardly ever met our business partners face to face, because they were in America and we were elsewhere. All the people in our support team were people I knew in the industry through these on-line networks.

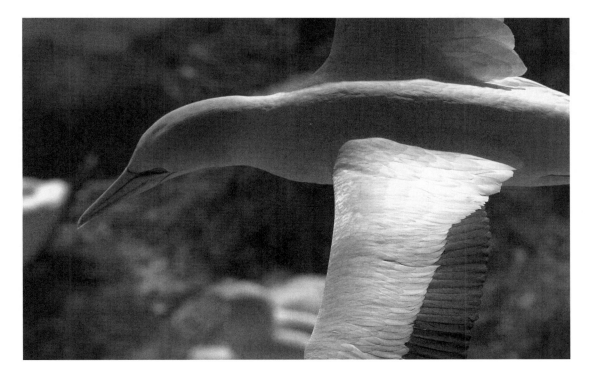

Then in the last year or two, there's been a profound shift in how things are happening, a coming of age of what we call Web-2.0, and that's about social networking on the web. This is where it's no longer the early adopters who love the technology, now it's mainstream. Every kid is on MySpace and YouTube. Everyone is blogging. You're seeing a shift even in how the media is happening. There are websites like Digg and Technorati, where you vote for cool pages you like, and those web pages can be authored by the individual, not big corporations. Then there's on-line dating. That's pretty popular too!

**Rose:** Yes, the Internet has opened up possibilities for global communication and co-creativity, bringing rapid evolutionary change into our lives. I'm interested in what you're doing now, Will.

**Will**: The journey I've been on these last two and a half years has shifted me internally and I'm very much in the heart space now. *Laughter.* All I want to do is service. I think of Buckminster Fuller and how he reached a point in his life where everything had gone wrong and he was about to jump off a bridge. As he gazed down from the bridge, he asked the question, "What would happen if I devote the rest of my life to the service of humanity?" From there, he went from everything in his life being in the pits of depression, to being a man with so much energy at eighty; he could devote his life to changing the world in his own unique way! I think of that often. I'm in this heart space, and the Art of Living advanced course with Sri Sri Ravi Shankar I've just returned from, is reinforcing that more and more. Yet at another level I know everything is an illusion!

**Rose:** What does it mean to you to serve humanity?

**Will:** It's getting back to the base of who we are. Everyone has that desire. When you ask children what they want to do when they grow up, answers are usually about service. For example, they want to be scientists so they can discover really cool things to help people. It was really clear to me as a kid that whatever else I wanted, I wanted to help people. Our basic nature, before all the complications come in, is about service to others. I think a daily practice is a really important part of that. In the entrepreneurial course Daniel and I ran, it came back to one thing: do you have a daily practice; something that gives you energy and will push you through the stressful hard times? From that energy, you do service, you do what your basic nature is. From that, you get more energy and it's an upwards spiral.

**Rose:** Your particular way of doing service is through technology?

**Will**: My passions are entrepreneurship and technology. My heart is helping and giving back. Combining the two, one is a fire and one is a feeling in the heart space. One is about having fun, and the other is feeling that deep fulfillment which sustains my soul.

*"Enlightenment is the journey from head
back to the heart, from words back to silence,
to innocence in spite of your intelligence."*

*" Life is sacred. Celebrate life.
Care for others and share whatever you
have with those less fortunate than you.
Broaden your vision for the
whole world belongs to you."*

—Sri Sri Ravi Shankar, Founder of The Art of Living

## We can change our minds

The recent movie, "The Secret", inspired millions of people to begin the practice of changing negative thought patterns into positive ones, in order to attract "what they want" into their lives. This teaching, based on the universal law of attraction, demonstrates how like energies attract each other. Negative thoughts create negative energy, which in turn attracts negative experience; whereas positive thoughts create positive energy and positive outcomes.

The skills for manifesting abundance presented in "The Secret": visioning, focus, intention, and practicing gratitude, are foundational to the art of conscious creating. As we develop this practice, we can go further and give more attention to the importance of balancing what the individual *wants* with what the collective *needs*, to make room for the "us" as well as the "me".

# *Shift Five*

## From relying on outer authorities to connecting instead with inner guidance, authentic values and creativity.

As we commit to self awareness, self knowledge and self responsibility, we learn to be present, listen inwardly and trust our intuition. As if by magic, everything we need for the next step of our learning "shows up", even though we may not always recognize it nor greet people or events with open arms. The synchronicities of life reveal an intrinsic harmony, which in turn may lead us to a deepening trust in, and curiosity about, the unfolding creative process of life.

# Frank Cook
## Here we are! Let's get to work!

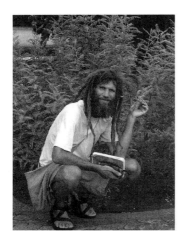

I travel most of the year teaching courses on Plant Spirit Medicine and Thrivalism. I have authored several books and am currently receiving my Masters in Holistic Science from Schumacher College in England. Over the last thirteen years, my passion for being a repository of plant knowledge has grown steadily. I have studied with herbalists, shamen, vaidyas, sangomas, green witches, doctors, professors, and medicine men around the world. They have initiated me into many ways of walking with plants. More and more, there are opportunities to share what I have learned at workshops, schools, conferences, and gatherings of all types. As an extensive traveller, I have developed a deep-rooted network of people whose lives are consciously intermingled with plants, healing, and ways to create a better world. I make a wide range of foods and medicines to share with my family, friends and community. I lead a simple life, communicating, teaching, reflecting, and spending a lot of time in the forests and gardens, delving deeper into the mysteries of the plant kingdom and our place in the web of life. I see us quickly becoming one world. My central questions in this respect are: what plants will be in our global gardens and stories? What will our global healing system look like? What are the roles of the human species in the web of life? Each of the cultures of the world has contributions to make. I intend to find out what they are and share these insights around the world, remembering that we come from Gaia; Gaia does not come from us. www.plantandhealers.com

**Frank**: Living my passion means not having to sacrifice or compromise myself in order to achieve my purpose here, and to look inside and find out why we're here, and live into it just as fully as I can.

**Rose:** It seems your passion is mostly focused around having a relationship with nature?

**Frank:** Yes, helping us humans recognize we're connected to nature. There's an illusion that's been going on now three or four hundred years in Western culture, that we are separate from nature. In the last hundred years, the consequences of this have accelerated to an incredibly fast rate, to the point we're living in bubbles or boxes basically. As much as we try to forget or pretend we're not part of nature, we certainly are. In that illusion of separation, we've really neglected our responsibility. It's coming back around now where the degradation of the environment is so huge, I think everyone has become aware of it at some level. We're realizing, "oh, there aren't as many birds as there were when I was a child " or "there aren't as many insects" or "I don't feel as healthy or strong as I did before", those kinds of things. What I'm interested in is how to take that personal awareness and apply it in our lives and our culture. I'm mostly talking about Western culture right now, and we're only 20% of the world. We really need to look out into the rest of the world, where people are still living in connection, as well as learning from our own journey of these last four hundred years.

**Rose:** Although, of course, the degradation of nature's going on throughout the world, isn't it?

**Frank:** Yes, the influences are everywhere. The veneer of Western modern living has its presence everywhere I've ever been. It's like a veneer spread over the Earth. Definitely the impact is huge! In some places that veneer is all encompassing, in other places it's just like a little outpost. Here in New Zealand, there are places that are very Western and very modern, and then places where you can get away from that and feel what was here before.

**Rose:** I've always felt the etheric body of the land is relatively intact here in Aotearoa, whereas in some places it's completely lost.

**Frank:** You can definitely feel, listening to the cicadas pulsing in the background, there's still a life vibrancy here the land is putting out, and that's so important, it's nature's wake-up call, nature saying 'hello!'

**Rose:** Do you feel a sense of mission to educate people into a better relationship with nature?

**Frank:** Oh definitely, mission is a good word. I think of myself as an evolutionary revolutionary! I've lived a relatively simple life, at least relative to the average Westerner, definitely not simple compared to the average person on Earth. Compared to some, I live like a king! This has given me a perspective of being able to recognize how much we can improve our lives if we get back to what's really important. It's definitely an everyday commitment. Every day is about how many people I can share and communicate with, to wake them up. That's why it's been so great hitchhiking around New Zealand because I've met a really neat collection of people. I've had forty-five rides and each one of them had its own special interaction. It was definitely part of my work to put out thoughts, listen and record, and this made my journey very meaningful.

**Rose:** Every synchronous meeting is an opportunity to be of service and to fulfill your mission!

**Frank:** Exactly, it *is* synchronous and it's great! The word coincidence has been co-opted. I think *co*-incidence has a very different meaning. *Co*-incidence means there's nothing random, everything's coming together. Some of these rides were like prearranged meetings, like "Here we are! Let's get to work!" I do fully believe the Universe meets you. It's an amazing, well, God, Great Spirit, or whatever words you want to use to describe That Which Is. It blows me away! It can be both Gaia and the whole world and these huge systems in which I'm just a little grain of sand, or it can be so personal it comes and literally whispers in your ear: "This is what you're here for!" Hitchhiking is a great reminder of that, because you really meet angels who are right there waiting to help you.

**Rose:** It's really a journey of trust?

**Frank:** It *is* and also a nice cleansing of my karmic field. I've had to reflect on all those hitchhikers I've passed on the road when I wasn't tuned in enough to stop and offer them a ride.

**Rose:** Is the ability to journey in trust something that's evolved for you? Do you feel you've always had that, or was there a certain moment when you woke up to all of this?

**Frank:** Yes, trust is definitely something that's had to come into fullness over the years. I don't know if I can think of one particular moment when all of a sudden I became trustful, but it's definitely how I live now. To get up the courage to really step out of the life I had been programmed and trained for, into the life I was really here to live, definitely involved the development of trust. I can remember the first hitchhiking I did, and the first time I ever ventured out of the familiar into the unknown. It's definitely complicated because in American society, the culture, in a sense, creates distrust. Despite all the propaganda about not trusting your neighbour, there are still people who are just beautifully trustful, who came along and picked me up. I'm amazed by that. I think it's our great hope that people still come from a place of trust and using their intuition.

**Rose:** I know you've travelled to many parts of the world and it seems that's bred hopefulness in you.

## Living a simple life

**Frank:** Yes, and we have to remember 80% of the world is not modern Western culture and most people live very, very simple lives. They use plants growing around them in daily life, in food, and in clothing. It's easy to forget how the majority of people on the planet live. We think everybody in the world is watching television and it's not true at all, about forty million viewers, that's all. Well shoot! That's a drop in the bucket compared to the numbers of us there are on the planet!

*Sam: A Caring Seed*

*If I could choose a seed for the base of a new world it would be caring. I choose caring because I strongly dislike anger in any form. The new world would have trees and plants everywhere. There would be no war, drugs or pollution; elegance would be a key factor in every part of life. People will love each other and help each other because they can, not because they will get something out of it.*

**Rose:** I think it's so important for us all to become simpler in the way we live. In my experience, trust has developed as I've shed conditioning and possessions. The more I do that, the greater the trust. I'm interested to hear what simplicity means in your life.

**Frank:** Well, wearing dreadlocks is a big one for me. I've just passed through twenty years of wearing dreadlocks! When they started growing I had no idea I was going to have them, I just stopped combing my hair. Over the years of having them I've asked, why do I have them, and why do I keep having them? Simplicity is probably one of the most important things they teach me. In the beginning, I just didn't need to be constantly doing myself up for society anymore. I wanted to get back to being who I simply am. Being who we are doesn't have to do with the clothes we wear or our material goods, nor with all these incredible systems of bank accounts, retirement plans, health insurance, that just box us into our little world and isolate us from the natural world.

In the States, at least in the middle class up, there's a sense of being raised to be the star of your own movie, and getting everyone else to be the supporting cast. It wasn't until the last five to ten years I started to realize, "Wait a minute! It's not my movie first of all, and I'm not the star of it, I'm just a participant. Here we are! How can I best be of service? What can I learn from this? What can I share in this?" I think a lot of it is getting out of the driver's seat of control, turning over control, surrendering, and letting things flow as best you can. There are some really virtuous people out there who have been models for that over the years and I fall way short of them. You saw by the size of my backpack, I still wield a bunch of weight. I still strive to keep gleaning out what I no longer need to be with me anymore and pass it on.

Also, in the States, there's a thing that doesn't get talked about and I'm sure it's true in a lot of places. When you get a job it's not just about having a job to get some money; there's an entire system you step into. Your self worth changes according to how much you're getting an hour or how much your time is worth. There's a mindset that takes you away from all the important things we're here to do, like connecting with nature. All of a sudden that apple tree full of apples in your back yard depreciates in value: "Oh, why would I go out and pick all those apples? I can go to the store. Three hours it takes to pick those apples, and box them up and make apple sauce. Three hours, that's $80. I could buy all the applesauce I want for that!" All of a sudden you've given your time, and other resources away preparing for work and coming down from work.

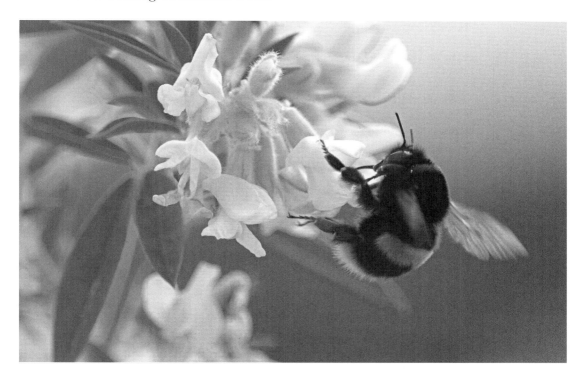

**Rose:** It's like stepping into time.

**Frank:** Yeah, we don't mean real time, we're talking about linear time which has been created by Greenwich Mean Time, with the arms of a clock going around. It's all a human construct, created to keep people working for the large system, measuring their time in dollars.

**Rose:** On the one hand, we have linear time, on the other we have what you might call participatory time. We let go of "the story-of-me" and step into "I'm just a participant" and that becomes a more co-creative dance.

**Frank:** Right, and it's not linear, it's a spiral! When you're meeting people, meeting plants, meeting the river, meeting the mountain, it's here we are again! What is it that's left over from the last time we were together? I can't remember the last time, but there's a feeling we've been here before! What's really important for me, and it's where a lot of my fuel comes in to give me the energy to teach and share, is whether people are really making a choice? Do they really have the spectrum of choice in front of them?

**Rose:** Conscious choice.

**Frank:** Yeah, conscious choosing.

## *The language of plants*

**Rose:** Going back to nature, you talk about plants as your friends. Do you feel you communicate with plants? Is that a language you're learning?

**Frank:** That's a good question, and it can be answered in all sorts of ways. I communicate with plants on many, many different levels. One of my teachers, Greenlight, talks about the language of all beings as a language that comes from the heart, not from the mind. There's a book by Stephen Harrod Buhner, *"The Secret Teachings of Plants"* that came out a year or two ago and has some fine teachings about how to use your heart to communicate with plants. By tuning into the vibes back and forth between the plant and you, your heart and your brain, you can figure messages and stories. There are many levels of that. My brain loves learning the knowledge of plants: who they are in relation to humans, who they are to themselves, their names, and how they relate evolutionarily.

Then there's another level of communication that's more subtle and kind of spectacular. Anyone can do this and one of the teachers I've had along the way, a woman called Starhawk, used to say, even if you don't get it right away, just play. Go up to a tree that calls out to you, it can be a special tree or a tree you just meet in the woods. Just go up and hug the tree, put your body as close to it as you can, wrap yourself around it as fully as you can, really just surrender to that tree with every bit of your being, even if it feels silly and awkward. Then say to the tree, "Tell me a story". It's amazing, it will always happen! You'll hear a story, and you may think your brain's telling it, but if you keep doing this, you're going to hear stories you never imagined. You're going to hear insights into things that you never thought about before. If you keep it up, you're going to realize these beings are sentient, vibrant, evolved, ancient and wise. There's a well-known book, *"Secret Life of Plants"*, which is an awesome book in many ways. All the experiments show how truly alive plants are! They move about! They have reactions! Plants are so much more remarkable than we think they are.

We eat, wear and use plants all the time, but it's not so much about using them. You wouldn't talk about using a human friend, that's not being very much of a friend. I want us to be friendlier with plants, have plant allies. I feel this way because of some of the work I've done over the years in spirit medicine; shamanistic work. I'm fascinated by that whole other level of communication where you come out of yourself, into the dream time, into other levels of consciousness, and you meet these beings in whole different ways. Their colours, vibrancy, and flavours communicate with me and teach me who they are.

Eat something wild every day! It doesn't have to be a whole plant, just nibble, and get to know the name and who it is. Susun Weed, a great herbalist in the States, said whatever you need most grows outside your back door. You'll meet a whole universe of beings coming up through the cracks! Really, we're here to be caretakers of the Earth. We have so many gifts and we've used these gifts in selfish, nonconnected ways. But the gifts are still there, and every day is an opportunity to plant seeds, to walk over and dig up a plant and replant it, or help a plant that's wounded. All these things are just calling out to us to step back into our role as guardians. The Cherokee talk about that in their history. Native American teachings have influenced me a lot. I guess they were the first voices I heard, outside my schooling, that encouraged me to come out of myself and start saying, wait a minute, there's something going on! It's nice the Maori have that wisdom here, that deep sense we come from the same place as the plants. The plants are our elders and we can learn from them. I'm really glad to find that in New Zealand. I find with all the indigenous cultures of the world, the obvious recognition we are connected, and that's a responsibility.

**Rose:** Maybe it starts with a bit of curiosity, or a desire to go out and have a look and see what's there, to look and listen?

**Frank**: Yes, every day is an opportunity to take those little steps and they start to increase, to build history, and all of a sudden you know the plants around you. Then you want to know more, so you just keep doing that. There are 325,000 plant species and a million species of insects. Wow! How many species of humans? Just one! I can't believe anyone is ever bored or at a loss what to do with their time. Just walk out the door, it's all there! And yes, simple curiosity, and desire for food, that's where I get a lot of people showing an interest. They want to know things they can eat, and then they're interested in aesthetics and the natural medicines. Plants are just there waiting to open up to friendship and relationship, to be allies. They're there for us. They're there to teach us. There's even a great argument plants created us because they needed somebody to help them move seeds!

**Rose:** We've evolved from them and they are incredibly abundant.

**Frank:** Abundance is really the way of Life. It's funny we've created an economic system that's about scarcity. One of my teachers at Schumacher College in England talked about really the only scarce thing in the world is money, and that's done on purpose to get people continuing to work. The truth is there's abundance. I was just at a plum tree the other day, and there were so many plums on just that one tree, I filled my pockets and ate all I could. If I lived nearby this tree, I'd be drying the plums or preserving the plums, all from the one little tree! There's so much out there: the seaweeds of the world and the wild mushrooms. I have to laugh when I hear people say there isn't enough food and there isn't enough medicine. It's our misperception that gets in the way. A lot of my writing comes from the desire to get people to recognize the sheer abundance of everything. The first principles of permaculture are to observe and interact. Interaction is the key. It can be little steps, it doesn't have to all happen in one day, but a little bit each day and you'll start to flow. What matters is recognizing the true abundance and participating in that abundance.

# Consciousness Is The Transformational Catalyst

Like the ancient art of alchemy, which changed base metal into gold, the process of transformation brings consciousness into form. It draws the invisible, formless, intelligent, universal life force, or spirit, into visible material actuality. As we participate in this process, we become co-creators with universal intelligence and enable "spirit" to move through us to express itself in the world of form. When we co-create with universal intelligence for the good of all, this is conscious evolution.

As we each make this choice to evolve consciously, we develop practices for maintaining higher consciousness by releasing old mental and emotional conditioning and pain held in the body. This letting go of old, limiting patterns of social conditioning creates more space in our minds, hearts, and bodies for the new consciousness, or universal intelligence, to flow through. This frees us to invent new forms of social organisation based on new cultural values. As we release whatever is keeping us heavy, muddled, opaque, blocked, and contracted, we become emotionally lighter, mentally clearer, more spacious, and more transparent, to ourselves and others. All the old conditioning is surrendered to the crucible of transformation: our "stories of me", our fixed beliefs about how the world is, the opinions we're attached to, and whatever else keeps us feeling separate, judging, and limited.

*What is the base metal in your life awaiting transmutation?*

*What in our social institutions is dull and heavy and longs for a catalytic spark to light the evolutionary fire?*

## The light and the dark

I was born in England in 1949. That makes me one of the "baby boomers" or "a child of the '60's". The sixties was an era of expansion, affluence, and optimism, following the horror and devastation of the Second World War and the austerity of the '50's. I think we were possibly the first generation to rebel en masse against the status quo. We wanted to change the world through a revolution of love, peace, free sexuality and expanded consciousness. It was the colourful beginning of a mass movement toward liberation, which has been evolving and playing itself out ever since. Part of that evolution has been in our understanding of what liberation means and how it is to be achieved.

Behind the celebration much darker realities loomed. As a teenager I first became aware of global politics, the threat of nuclear weapons, and the fragility of life on Earth. I carried the image of a man in a gray suit with his finger poised carelessly over a button which could release nuclear fire and poison into the world. Of course, this had already happened in Hiroshima. I was blooming into young womanhood and this spectre of annihilation was a blight on the rose. This has been a motivating force in my life ever since. I have lived with the awareness that life on Earth hangs in the balance and the way our global society is organized is far from just, allowing far from a full expression of human potential. Yet despite the darker aspects of humanity, I have always felt privileged to be alive at this time and I have always known there was some unique contribution for me to make; that becoming more conscious matters. This has made for an interesting life.

It seems to me, it is this interplay between the dark and the light that characterises our age. We evolve through this tension. Maybe it has always been so, yet the stakes are much higher now, aren't they? I believe this is the first time in the history of humankind we have had the ability to destroy each other and our environment on a global scale. Are we such a sleepy species that we have had to take ourselves to the brink of annihilation to wake ourselves up? What a peculiar dilemma we find ourselves in: an archetypal battle between the forces of dark and the forces of light, the bad guys versus the good guys and none of us know whether we will live to tell the tale. How do we make sense of this? Is it time to write ourselves a new myth, to embrace a new cosmology, grow a new culture?

## *The expansion of consciousness*

The evolution of consciousness is inextricably interwoven with social history, the unfolding of culture and the events of our daily lives. Jean Gebser, Swiss cultural philosopher whose magnum opus, "The Ever-Present Origin", was published in 1949 and 1953, was considered an Einstein of the consciousness movement. He said the best way to understand consciousness is to look for the patterns in the daily events of our lives, rather than developing ideas about consciousness and then applying them to what we see. This has always been my preferred way too, to start from experience and move towards theory.

It's been fascinating watching the wild ride of history unfolding during my nearly sixty years of life on Earth. Consciousness has expanded in every direction: deep into the inner world, far into outer space. It has infused the social world, drawing people together in social liberation movements and bringing to a head seemingly irreconcilable difference between nations. In both personal and collective life, consciousness nudges abuses, secrets, and lies to the surface to be healed. It ushers in radical change, expansion, chaos, destruction, time pressure, exponential complexity, confusion and interconnectedness. Within this evolution of consciousness, the individual is a holon or microcosm of the whole; the whole can only evolve through the individual.

Can we track the evolution of consciousness in our own lifetime? To attempt to do so in a few paragraphs is a risky venture, yet as I identify some of the strands of evolving consciousness I have been aware of in my lifetime, I hope they will touch your own memories, and demonstrate how complex is this interweaving of evolving consciousness through personal and collective life.

## *The personal is political*

In the '60's psychedelics exploded into popular culture within a renaissance of music, creativity and the cult of youth. Many stumbled unconsciously into previously unknown and spectacular inner dimensions. For some, the realization of the multi-dimensional nature of reality led to more sober explorations of inner space through the practice of meditation, the study of Eastern philosophies and pilgrimages to Indian gurus; bringing East and West together in a new way. Alongside these new frontiers of consciousness, emerged the Civil Rights movement, the Women's Liberation movement, and the anti-nuclear movement. "The personal is political" became our mantra. People were on the move, and the world began to open up, with global travel becoming affordable to many for the first time. The first humans landed on the moon and sent back the very first pictures of our beautiful blue/green planet revolving in space. My brother, David, returning home from work one day, brought the news the computer he was working with was as big as a room. This was the first time I had ever heard of a computer!

## *Group consciousness raising*

In the '70's we witnessed beginning concerns about exploitation of the environment and birthed the Environmental movement. Petrol prices started to rocket, at least where I was living in the UK. The anti-nuclear movement became more vociferous against the proliferation of nuclear power, and the short and long term implications of where, and how, to dump poisonous nuclear waste came to the fore. Feminists formed consciousness-raising groups, developing a collective process to examine how the oppressive and divisive mores of a culture are passed on through the psyche of the individual. Humanistic psychology gave birth to existential therapies like Gestalt, Psychodrama, and Transactional Analysis, and body therapies such as Bio-Energetics, and these became widely available and affordable to middle income earners. In both the inner and the outer world, consciousness was expanding, and it wasn't always comfortable nor regarded as positive.

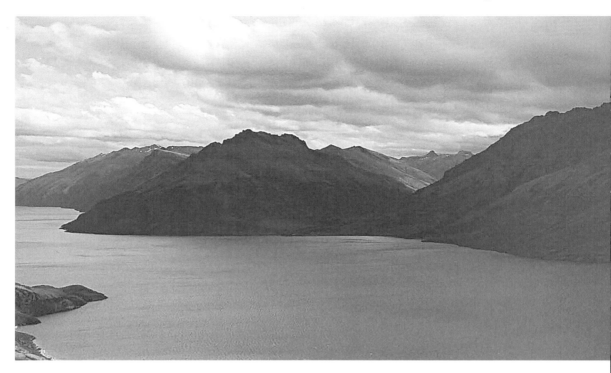

## *Cynicism, spin and falling walls*

In the '80's, there was a deepening cynicism in the body politic, an accelerated destruction of the natural world, and the outbreak of the AIDs epidemic. Growing numbers joined the consciousness trail through psychotherapy, personal growth workshops, meditation practices and alternative health care. The omnipresence of television meant global news travelled fast and much of it was bad news. The "Live Aid" concert in 1985 joined millions of people around the world for the first time in a celebration of rock music whilst raising awareness and funds for famine relief in Ethiopia. The Harmonic Convergence in August 1987 brought news of the Mayan prophecy and our approach to the end of time, and was heralded by many as the beginning of the New Age, the Age of Aquarian group mind. The '80's went out with a bang when the Berlin Wall fell in November 1989 and the end of the Cold War marked the dissolution of the USSR. Just as sudden and surprising was the release from prison of Nelson Mandela and the beginning of his new life as an ambassador of peace in a deeply divided South Africa,

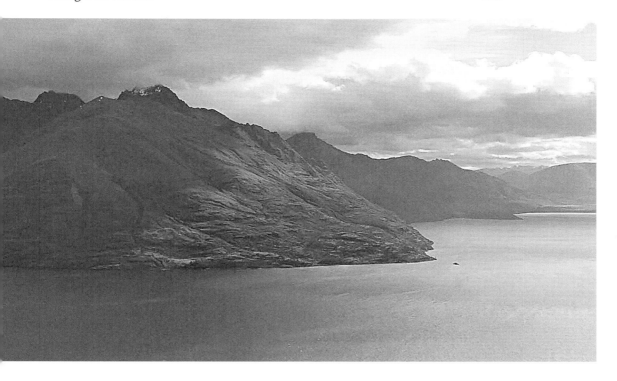

in 1990. Yet the dissolution of old forms and oppressive regimes gave birth to greater complexity and new social problems.

## *Preparing for Y2K*

Maybe this was the beginning of the big global meltdown, yet few governments were taking environmental issues seriously. In 1990, conflict in the Middle East escalated when the United Nations entered Iraq in the Gulf War. The '90's saw technological revolution sweeping the world, with computers in every home and many five years olds more computer-literate than their parents. The impending technological crisis Y2K never came, but it did raise the alert for a possible crash of global life support systems. Meanwhile the Internet quietly revolutionized the world, seamlessly knitting us into one and a revolution in physics uncovered the emptiness of form. For the first time in many centuries, science and spirituality began to merge in the understanding we inhabit a universe which is essentially energy-in-motion.

Against this cultural backdrop, growing numbers of people became more seriously committed to exploring consciousness through spiritual paths, both ancient and modern. For many, at least at first, this was a path of personal liberation, with the goal of enlightenment. New Age beliefs and practices for "manifesting an abundant reality" grew alongside the seasoned traditions of Yoga, Buddhism and the Perennial Wisdom, and some formed bridges between the ego-strengthening work of psychotherapy and the ego-release of spirituality.

Billions of people around the world partied on 31st December 1999, ready to bring in a new millennium and a new era. This marked the end of a century notable for barbaric acts of humans towards their own kind, and gross acts of savagery towards the natural world. Amidst the chaos and profound political cynicism, there started to emerge a vision of One World and One Global Family.

## Catastrophic new beginnings and the way of the bodhisattva

### Lauren: A Caring Seed

*If I can sow a seed for a new world it would be caring. Everything would be bright and colourful and there would be happiness everywhere. Everything would be clean and there would be no more littering. There would be buildings in all shapes and sizes. There would be no more bullying or arguing because everybody would act like family. I think it is the best virtue and I would love to live there.*

As we headed into the first years of the 21st century catastrophe followed catastrophe: 9/11, mad cow disease, tsunamis, bird flu, hurricane Katrina, an earthquake in Pakistan, war in Iraq, religious fundamentalism, the oil crisis, and global warming, to name a few. More and more people began to wake up to the realization there is no individual salvation. There is no Paradise outside of all this, no freedom we can escape into, no one to whom we can pass the buck. This is it! We are it!

It is this realization of our essential interconnectedness and the personal responsibility which arises from compassion for the human condition, which I understand to be the calling of the present day bodhisattva. One of my teachers, Joanna Macy, described it thus:

*The bodhisattva, the Buddhist hero figure, is one who knows and takes seriously the dependent co-arising of all things. That is why he also knows that there is no private salvation, and that is why she turns back from the gates of nirvana to reenter samsara, the world of suffering, again and again, to minister to all beings until each, to every blade of grass, is enlightened. Here is revealed the compassion which blooms naturally when we open to our condition of profound mutuality. Since that condition pertains to all of us, whether or not we acknowledge it yet, we are all, in a sense- the Scripture tells us – bodhisattvas.*

## Balancing negative energy

It is all pretty overwhelming when we stop to consider the world we're living in and how complex life has become. There is an enormous challenge in maintaining a state of consciousness that does not escape into denial and yet remains positive. I experience this challenge every day.

I truly believe our global crisis is a crisis of perception and consciousness. The ways we are conditioned to perceive reality causes problems, not reality itself. Our perceptions are coloured by our beliefs, values, emotional states and states of mind, or in other words our states of consciousness. Choosing to develop and maintain consciousness in higher states is a form of service. More spiritual teachers are suggesting that environmental pollution mirrors the pollution in our own minds. Violence and wars, as well as peace, begin in our relationships with self, with each other, and with all beings. More and more people are recognizing that creating a better world starts with a daily consciousness practice. In line with the acclaimed writers on consciousness, David Hawkins and Ken Wilber, and avatars of the Oneness Blessing Amma and Baghavan, Anahata and Orah propose that higher states of consciousness balance negative energy in our environment. MSI, the enlightened founder of the Society for Ascension said it will take only 64.000 enlightened individuals to balance the negative energy in the world, to lift collective consciousness into a greater appreciation of our interconnectedness and safeguard Life on Earth.

## *Finding a common language for inner experience*

Finding a language for inner experience helps the discovery of shared understandings and meanings for human life, and the exploration of the higher purpose of life on Earth. This seems a very important focus of our consciousness work. Shared language, meanings, values, and stories contribute to building a new culture and support everyone involved. Dialogue and deeper conversations can be wonderfully exciting forums for this process of discovery. When such conversations happen in larger groups and from a state of presence, they create containers in which we can move collectively beyond the limitations of individual thought, into the unknown empty space of limitless creative possibilities, synergy and co-creation.

The next four interviews are personal explorations of the spiritual journey. Each person shares his or her own individual experiences of moving in their own unique way towards unity consciousness. This is a state of mind in which the Oneness of all life has been realized, through connection with the essential self. I find these interviews exciting. Many people are moving into hitherto unknown states of consciousness and attempting to make sense of their experience. These interviews offer slices of life from a few people who engage with these questions of consciousness on a daily basis, and for whom growing in consciousness is their passion.

**John Massey:** One of the many things I like about this interview is the deliberation with which John develops his spiritual understandings. No beliefs are simply swallowed whole, everything is tested through experience, and ideas worked through until they make complete sense to him, and can be fully owned. He explores his understanding of human separation from nature as a disconnection from our inner essence. To connect with essence is to connect with the wholeness and harmony of nature. For John, establishing a daily rhythm supports this connection as he progresses towards the realization of unity.

**Mirjam Busch and Rudolf Jarosewitsch:** My intention was to talk with Mirjam and Rudolf about conscious relationship, a process which holds core skills necessary for humanity's transition to the new culture. However Mirjam was in a new and unknown space, of great relevance to the subject of consciousness, and we immediately leapt into conversation about that. She recounts very clearly how it feels to be in the middle of a transformational shift when lifelong patterns are being shed and identity itself is changing. By contributing so openly from her inner life, she helps build a shared "map of the territory". As we journey into new states of consciousness, knowing how to support ourselves in the unknown, in spaciousness and presence, is vitally important for our evolution. Rudolf explores how becoming more true to himself, presents the challenge of differentiation in relationship. Through the practice of conscious relationship, he and Mirjam learn how to allow and value their differences.

**Jonathan Evatt:** For me, this interview is a wonderful example of how dialogue can unfold when two people stay present to the arising moment. It extended my understanding of how universal intelligence works through us, by challenging us to bring forth more of our personal power and open to a more spacious, more inclusive identity, as spiritual beings. When we live at the unfolding edge of consciousness, at the borderland with the unknown, we expand the known by shining the light of consciousness into the unknown within ourselves, giving expression to it, and integrating it into a more inclusive perception of reality. As our collective "known" breaks down we are faced with the challenge of learning to live with the unknown and trust in our creative powers.

**Anahata and Orah Ishaya** describe their process of spiritual awakening and quest for Oneness, initially through immersion in the spiritual community of the Ishaya's Ascension, and then through becoming givers of Deeksha, the Oneness Blessing.

## *There is an evolutionary intelligence moving through us*

Living through this transitional moment in humanity's history can be very uplifting and certainly stressful, even terrifying at times. There is a point in the creative process when the new is very close to manifesting and the strain of holding and containing the creative energy becomes almost too much to bear. As we move more fully into the storm of global transformation, perhaps you sense an evolutionary intelligence moving through you more urgently? Do you feel a creative force drawing you out, calling to you, compelling you to move? Has your old way of life become intolerably suffocating? Have you noticed how time appears to be alternately speeding up or slowing down? Maybe you're very busy, feeling focused, energized and purposeful, and then you drop into a more contracted, lower energy state, as old pain or fear surfaces to be processed? Could this be the cosmos fulfilling its destiny through you? Pulsing through you? Giving birth to itself through you? Clearing away everything in its path that does not serve consciousness? Making you a vessel for global transformation?

## *What does living your passion mean to you?*

*The spiritual work I do is to find a rhythm with nature that works for me in relationship to the whole. I believe we're actually working toward unity and that means aspiring to our individualised highest level of divinity. —John*

*To give myself permission to really enter into the not knowing and not have to fix it or fill it with meaning and solutions, I think this is the seedbed. I really feel I am preparing the ground for my true passion to flourish. —Mirjam*

*For me, it has to do with conscious partnership and compassionate communication. I tie it into the challenge of differentiation. I think it's an ongoing challenge in every relationship: how can you be your individual self and be in relationship? —Rudolf*

*The Universe is always presenting me with a challenge as it manifests through me from moment to moment. Living my passion is about remaining present with the challenge that's forever presenting itself in many different forms. —Jonathan*

*The passion of getting to know God really came to me in full force. I heard my girlfriend say: "Well you know we're all One, don't you?" That totally changed my life. That one sentence took me out of one world and shifted me into another°! All of a sudden, my brain and my heart and my being went: "What is this? What's this all about? I have to know!" From then on, it was a continuous search for Oneness. It became my beacon and I followed it like a moth to a flame. —Anahata.*

*I've realized it's not an individual journey; it has to be a collective thing. The desire has changed to one of wanting everybody to experience unity. Ultimately, the goal is to experience causeless joy and love. —Orah*

# Shift Six

**From an illusion of separation and a belief we have to "do it alone" to a realization we are participating in an intelligent, abundant and friendly universe, which is calling us to be of service to the whole.**

Becoming more inwardly satisfied, and consciously focused on creativity, we experience at a deeper level the interconnected web of consciousness that runs through all life. As we develop acceptance and love of our own nature, the profound abundant generosity of life is revealed.

# John Massey
## Finding unity within stillness

John Massey lived his early life amongst a more tradi-tional farming community, but having been influenced by the desire to live differently on and with the land, through the 60's, 70's, and 80's, he became very involved with organic farming practices, particularly in horticulture. He worked for over twenty years with Community Gardens, mainly in the north of the South Island of New Zealand, as a coordinator and teacher. John's interest in, and passion for, organic gardening, are influenced by his study and practice of Yoga and his study of ancient wisdom. His vision is in understanding

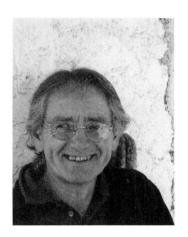

and working more intuitively with nature in ways that will help him and others live more harmoniously on the Earth. John runs courses on "practical herbalism" in Golden Bay, sharing ways of relating more harmoniously to the Plant Kingdom. He also works as a holistic pulser and massage therapist, bringing into his healing modalities his strong earth connec-tion. He is a yoga teacher and support person to an autistic man. John is currently involved with esoteric study groups and Compassionate Nonviolent Communication (CNVC) groups, and is studying esoteric healing. John's meditational work is related to his connection with these groups, and through this collective focus, grounding or anchoring the spiritual into daily living.

The first time I met John he was cooking "soul food" for a Soul Retreat in Totaranui, Golden Bay. I was amazed he could produce such good food from such simple ingredients. A few years later, together with

Robina, we returned to the same stunning location in the Abel Tasman National Park, for the first Earth Spirit Nature Retreat. I was struck by the patient, detailed attention John gave to plants and people alike. Later we co-created the first experiment in Soul Sanctuary, an adventure in group dialogue. It seems he has always been there as someone with whom I could share soulful conversations.

## *Exploring the wholeness of nature*

**Rose:** Would you like to jump in at the deep end, John, and say what living your passion means to you?

**John:** Well, this idea of living my passion is something that's evolving for me, because it relates to the unfolding nature of being. I am an explorer by nature and I think we are all explorers in one way or another. We have this mind, you see, that is continually probing. It wants to know why we are here, who we are, and where we might be going, if indeed we are going somewhere.

Part of my work or passion then, is to explore what, or how, my relationship to nature might be. I'm not the only one exploring that, because others write or talk about, either humanity's disconnection from nature, or what it means to be reconnected.

Some of my work is to take people into the natural world of gardens, cultivated or uncultivated. We learn about the plant kingdom mostly, and its relationship to the Earth and other beings. I find generally people want to know about the plants. They want information, such as how a particular plant is useful to us humans. The essence I believe, is just to be still and connected, and the plants will reveal their higher truth to the quiet mind.

In our human world there is so much movement, and so much information available, that being still, physically and mentally, is one of our greatest challenges. I wish to discover the peace and stillness within, the essence that simultaneously connects me to the wholeness of nature. In this place there is no separation. It is a constant journey of exploration or rediscovery, and there is a need just to be patient with it.

**Rose**: Do you think we people from Western culture have become alienated from nature?

**John:** Yes, I do. Even though people connect with nature on some levels, we're still disconnected overall. There's a huge war against nature in the way we live, and in our attitudes. The term terrorism is very common in people's minds these days. I see huge acts of terrorism against nature. It happens in the oceans, in the rain forests, and in people's gardens. The way we live, driving around in cars or building fences causes a big separation. That's partly because we're not at ease within and that means we are separated from the Higher Self, or the soul, which in truth is the real being.

**Rose:** So there's a connection between who we really are and nature?

**John:** Absolutely! Once we're really connected with our inner or Higher Self, with soul, whatever you want to call that, there's no division. Collectively, we're in the process of rediscovering this at the moment. Part of the problem is we have to "make a living", and generally that seems to take us away from nature. We focus on our self-centred human existence and how we can best live on the Earth, and take from the earth, rather than how we can live in harmonious relationship with the Earth and all creatures. It's quite a juggle to be harmonious with nature, and with human beings, within the social system that's been created.

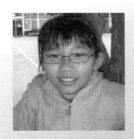

*Jenny: A Friendly Seed*

My *WHOLE NEW WORLD* seed would be a friendly, peaceful, and lovable seed. The seed starts off with a colorful heart-shaped seed and it will grow into a new planet where everyone is equal. There will be no cultural prejudice against anyone. People will share, and weapons and violence will be destroyed. Everyone would have a happier life.

**Rose:** So you're saying to be harmonious with nature we need to be harmonious with the Higher Self. This in itself is quite a challenge! How do we learn to live in inner peace?

**John**: The spiritual work I do involves finding a rhythm with nature that works for me in relationship to the whole. My own pathway is quite solitary at times, and I think that's what's needed sometimes, because in that solitariness it's possible to connect with Higher Self and with nature. Eventually the journey goes full circle because the relationship or connection with Higher Self also connects one to everyone and everything.

**Rose**: Do you think it's essential to be solitary to connect with Higher Self?

**John**: At certain times, yes. Once that connection's really established you never lose it amongst other people. Whereas, before that connection's well established, it's easy to lose it amongst others, because there's such a flow of energy between humans. Our culture is personality and lifestyle centred, and one gets easily drawn into that.

**Rose:** I'm inquiring into the possibility that what we're really connecting with is a universal intelligence, or consciousness, which runs through everything: through self, through nature, and through cosmos. Yet, as you say, with the lifestyle most people lead, there are many things to distract us from "tuning in" to universal intelligence, so we mostly exist in a more dualistic, time bound state of mind.

**John:** I think humanity is heading to a place of reconnection and there's a sense we need to do it quickly. I don't think we can do this very quickly; we have to be patient and take each step. There may be shortcuts, a quantum leap in consciousness perhaps, otherwise we just keep going on with the goal in mind. It's quite difficult to stay focused, because our daily needs seem more important than a higher goal. From a yogic point of view, what we're trying to achieve is having, or knowing, unity. I'm still figuring out what that means. I believe it means a known unity with all things, but sometimes, with all the focus on the disharmony in the world, it's hard to hold a sense of developing unity. Nevertheless, I think that's where we're headed. We have to keep that goal of unity in mind and keep going step by step.

## Finding a rhythm

**Rose:** Could you tell us a little about your own journey towards reconnection and unity? What has that involved and what have you learned?

**John:** Well, I started out not really knowing what it was I was meant to be doing. I had a difficult, problematic childhood, but I see now those challenges set me up to be more introspective and searching, and were actually quite useful in making me more understanding about things. My pathway for the search took me around the world. It was the '60's,' 70's and '80's and I was, like many others, in a time of great change and trying to find what was meaningful. During that time, I connected with the alternative movement and also knowingly began my spiritual development. Now, as I continue through my life, I find I'm getting deeper and deeper into spiritual practice, and it's about going towards unity.

**Rose:** When you talk about spiritual practice, what is yours? What does it involve?

**John:** It involves a study of spiritual texts and current enlightened writings, and a regular discipline like meditation, which for me, is a Yoga practice. It's not just yoga for the physical body. The practice is concerned with refining or training the mind and body, so they become vehicles for the soul. If I want to develop spiritually, I have to have rhythm in my life. I certainly need and respond to that. It's not just about putting aside work time and the need to make money, although that can be a spiritual practice too, but making time to do things that really nurture my Higher Self. The mind is trained to gradually get a perspective on what it is I really, really want. Through the training and rhythmic living, I get a clearer and more focused perspective on what a spiritual practice really is.

**Rose:** Would you say what you really want is this sense of unity?

**John:** Yes, a sense of unity and peace of mind.

**Rose:** Yoga is a pathway to that?

**John:** For me it is. It's a daily rhythmic discipline that keeps me focused, and in the discipline or practice, I am guiding my mind and body towards unity. I teach yoga, and I'm also involved with an Internet study group on aspects of Raja Yoga, (yoga of the mind). I sense we're all searching for the same thing and it's interesting, it's partly through technology we're able to link with others who are doing the same sort of work to develop this idea of unity. We don't have to be living next to one another to be connected!

I'm aware there's a gradual sense of unity developing on one level in the human family, yet on another level, there's still a great sense of disharmony, separation, difference, and an attitude of us-against-them. This is still obvious in the media, but I think the work I, and other people who are spiritually involved do, is gradually changing that disharmony. I sense a shift in consciousness developing. The spiritual focusing can lead towards inner peace and more understanding, which can then hopefully radiate out and affect human consciousness more widely. Energy follows thought. It's really important we aim, or focus, on the work of consciousness raising.

**Rose:** How does your practice help you in terms of day-to-day living? Have you noticed your relationships have changed through doing this work? Has it become easier to relate to other people?

**John:** Yes, it does help me, as long as I can stay really grounded. This means continuing to do my daily practices, having rhythm in my life, and also connecting with nature. It's a very holistic thing. When all these aspects are present, I can connect more deeply with myself and with others. With all the changes going on right now in the world, such as climate change, it takes quite a lot to maintain equilibrium. I believe these changes to the Earth's environment affect us; we humans are not separate from environmental changes but part of the Earthly environment. I sense there is something similar to climate change going on within us, different from personal health issues. We can't help but be affected by what we know, through the media and science, and by what we feel.

**Rose:** All the changes in society put us under pressure and, on the other hand, there are changes happening to the Earth. As individuals, we're, in a sense, caught between these forces and having to keep some personal balance, equilibrium and peace of mind within that. This is a huge challenge in itself!

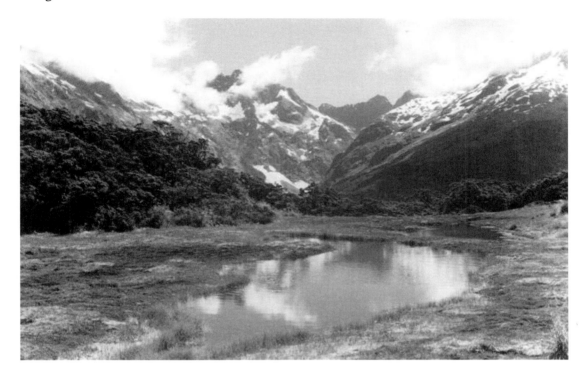

## *A Greater Plan?*

**John:** It is a huge challenge, and that's why it's important to keep developing a focus on, if you want to call it God, or our Higher Nature. Personally, it's a bit more difficult because I don't have a living Master, a living guide. I haven't been drawn to that. I have to keep seeking the essence, if you like, of life or nature, through an eclectic way, developing the idea of an overall guiding force, and how I can link with that. I know there is something that we fit into, some overall scheme or plan. My reading suggests, or refers to, the "Plan for Humanity" and the unfolding of the nature of Earth, or the unfolding of Nature. Most people can focus on a personal plan or goal but the idea of a greater plan is too much. I'm trying to get a perspective on the "Greater Plan"; I'm a bit foggy about what that is, but the more I keep working with it, the more it develops. If I really look at what's happening globally, I can see we are developing towards a "Greater Plan". Everything is unfolding towards some point: wars, tragedy, famine, death, these are all forms of change; an evolution that leads us towards some different way of being. The great thing is we can co-create our destiny. I believe we are doing that and our ability to communicate more efficiently is helping immensely.

**Rose:** Can you say something about what that destiny might be?

**John:** Once again, it's about finding unity. I believe we're actually working towards that, and unity means aspiring to our highest individualised level of divinity. There is, in that place, more unity than on the level of the personality.

**Rose:** Do you see this particular time as being pivotal?

**John:** Yes, I do.

**Rose:** The way I understand it is, we're in a portal at the moment, a time of opportunity, and it's not necessarily preordained how it will all unfold, or what the result will be.

**John:** I do think it's a pivotal time, a time of transformation. It's also a chaotic time, because in order to move forward we have to let go of attachment to things, and attachment to the self-serving personality, and that's quite difficult! In order to have more unity with everyone, and with nature, and with the Higher Self, there has to be a great degree of simplification. We can't have unity if there's too much going on in our minds and so much baggage from the past holding us back. I believe we're required to live more simply, and not only clear the mind, but focus it. That means letting go of a lot of "stuff", such as old beliefs. This doesn't mean to say I don't have "things" at all, but I learn to become unattached to things. For my own sense of well-being there is quite a transformation to go through, like a portal of new understanding or change in consciousness. This doesn't happen all at once, although it may do so for some. It's also about letting go of attachment to one's own well-being, in terms of the tendency to be completely self-serving. There are many paradoxes with this. We still have to look after our physical bodies, but not to the extent we're not looking after everything else.

## Seeing everything exactly as it is

I've been getting involved with NVC, Nonviolent Communication, and there's a large group coming together here in Golden Bay. A lot of people want to do this work, which is basically learning about one's own wants and needs, by really defining what they are. If you ask a lot of people what they want, they don't really know. I feel this is an integral part of the development of the human culture. In the end, I think it's about unity/harmony with self and right relationship with everything. This movement shows me there's lots of progress going on in human evolution. It's a small part, but it's really instrumental.

The practice of nonviolent communication includes developing the skills of observation and awareness, so when we're interrelating with any being, we're acknowledging what it is that being really wants or needs, without being critical or judgmental in any way. As we develop skills of observation we find clarity in seeing everyone exactly as they are and everything exactly as it is. In my work with nature, I teach people about connecting with medicinal plants or herbal plants, and this seeing everything exactly as it is, is important here too. People have difficulty with it, because it's the nature of the human mind to want to know the value of things. They want to know what everything is, and how it works. Yet when we step aside from that wanting, we see everything as it actually is, and then we know something greater! There's another paradox in there.

**Rose:** Yes, when you're really present with something, you know it without trying to name it, label it, control it, or understand it.

**John:** Exactly, it is about being present.

## Training the mind

**Rose:** When I'm present, say with a tree, I can start to feel its presence. Then there can be a communication between my presence and its presence, which is actually the same presence. Is this what you mean?

**John:** Yes, that's right. There's a need for discipline in training the mind to develop clarity and stillness. That's where a practice comes in, a physical, mental, or meditation practice, to develop that one-pointedness, which then overflows into everything. It's very gradual, and it's very important to do it on a daily basis, not just to practice physical yoga, but to practice the skills of stillness, observation and mindfulness.

**Rose:** It's also about seeing through the layers of mind, which prevent us from seeing, or being with, something or someone.

**John:** We've come through a period of time using the mind to discover things, to make things particular and see how things are put together. I think an aspect of human nature has become rather obsessive with that.

**Rose:** An analytical model: you pull things apart?

**John:** Yes, various writings talk about that. It's the nature of the human mind to want to know about things and there's nothing wrong with that. We also have to let go of some of the need to be particular and learn to see everything as a whole and the relationships between the parts. We're obviously in relationship with everything, because every-thing's living. It's all working in a kind of unity. Separation, as I see it, is just in the human mind and the goal is to try and find the way back to unity, through working on the mind to change attitudes and patterns of belief.

**Rose:** When people come to Golden Bay for the Earth Spirit Nature Retreat, they are immersed in nature for a week or more. Are they resistant, at some level, to being in nature or is there more a sense of a great relief and joy?

**John:** There seems to be a great relief and joy. However, as facilitators, we're still discovering within ourselves how to develop a real connec-tion to nature. Sometimes we get to the end of the Earth Spirit Nature Retreat and find we're just actually beginning! We still have a sense of busyness, of doing things. Really, all we need to do is be still, and in that stillness, make contact with the greater mind of Nature. Often people aren't quite ready to jump into that stillness straight away, because they're so used to being busy.

**Rose:** Do you think stillness is threatening to people?

**John:** It's the nature of the human mind to want to be busy, to be doing something. There's another paradox in there! The evolutionary nature of life just keeps moving forward and we're part of that. For example, I'm hungry so I have to get something to eat. I either have to grow food or make money to buy it, and that creates an impetus to keep moving. Or, I want to know something, so I look on the Internet to find out about it. I have to work. I have to be involved with something. There's a calling to work with, or be amongst, or with other people. I can't just be still continually. Sitting still is contradictory to the evolutionary nature. I have to keep interacting with life. People keep moving. Everything keeps moving. To be still within daily life is tricky and challenging but I think in reality, stillness is a state of mind; it's not just a state of not moving.

**Rose:** The Earth Spirit Nature Retreat offers people the opportunity to step out of busy life into a stiller space, yet even within that retreat space, it's difficult to get away from being busy!

**John:** Yes, sometimes we have to step out of things in order to see them clearly. It's helpful sometimes to step out of the structure of the life we're involved in, whether that's one's personal life, the life within a nation, or the life within the world; to step out, to see clearly, and then step back in, holding that clarity as we re-engage.

**Rose:** Maybe that's what a retreat can offer: a place where people can step out of everyday life, and then step back in with a new perspective? With the world getting busier and more chaotic, retreats could be a safety mechanism.

**John:** Yes, it is important to have retreats to get that clear perspective. Retreats offer many things: a change of perspective, steadiness and harmony, calmness, and insights into living. There's something in the human psyche that wants to put things right, to fix oneself or somebody else, yet we get confused about how to do that. This is where one wants to practice being clear and observing without making judgments.

**Rose:** Without trying to interfere! For me, the opposite of interfering is participating with, or co-creating with, being alongside something and flowing with it, rather than trying to control it and impose my own direction onto it.

## Self healing organisms

**John:** Life has the ability to maintain itself. A human organism, or the Earth for that matter, has the ability to find equilibrium, given the chance. When a human being is ill, s/he will often, given a chance to rest, regain equilibrium. In the healing modalities I practice, I find there is such a temptation to interfere and want to make things better. But it's not that simple. If someone has a physical or emotional problem, it didn't occur just a few minutes ago. It's been there for a long time. A person has to do a lot of their own personal work, once again, changing patterns. I think this wanting to make things better is pretty prevalent in the human mind. You can see it with the global situation. We think we have to make things better. Probably what we need to do is counteract the things which are harmful to the Earthly environment. We are starting to do that slowly, but we are still entrenched in ideas of self satisfaction.

**Rose:** Do you think with the way things are now, with the imbalances humanity has created in nature, the Earth can regenerate itself?

**John:** I've no doubt about that. The Earth as an organism is changing. If we get the human mind out of the way, it will heal itself, and it just may do that in ways unacceptable to us humans. We talk about nature as life on Earth, but Nature's much bigger than that. It's everything! We have to remember that. Maybe things happening on Earth are reflecting changes within our planetary system, and even beyond, in the universal system. People are saying humans are responsible and, of course, we are responsible to a point, but there are other big changes going on, interplanetary or inter-universal, that could be affecting what's happening on Earth. I don't think this global climate change is a one-time event; I 'm sure the Earth has gone through major changes many times.

**Rose:** We need to be humble in the face of all this.

**John:** Yes, but it doesn't mean we don't have to do anything! We do have to do things and we are doing things. I find it encouraging the global situation is bringing people together. We have to do something towards healing, although not necessarily healing the planet. I think the healing is needed in our relationships with each other and with all creatures. If we could do that, the healing and well-being of the Earth will automatically follow. Healing begins in the individual, and spreads out from the heart, and in the end, we do it all together. This is where something like nonviolent communication comes in. Through this work, people are learning to listen to one another, and there is healing in that.

There is a crisis, and through crisis, we move forward. You were talking about moving through a portal. A time of crisis is a portal, a time to move forward. It is well known that crises in people's lives are opportunities to move forward, so the crisis that's happening in humanity is an opportunity to move forward and come together in a different way.

*Project Port Lyttelton, Seven Oaks. Setting up a two acre organic garden growing produce and providing education on sustainable matters for the Lyttelton community – some of workers sharing a break.*

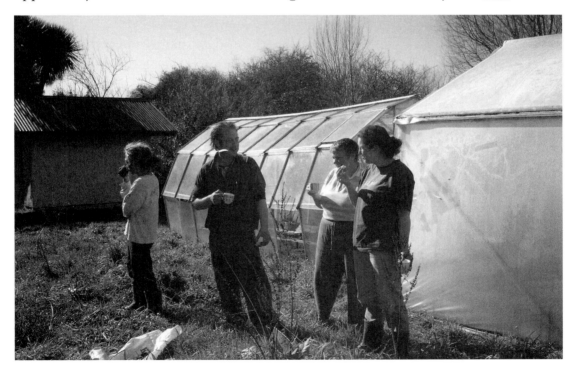

**Rose:** As you're talking, I'm seeing these two great forces: nature, on one hand, and society on the other. It seems the crisis we're in, is an opportunity to harmonise these two aspects; to create a culture which brings society into relationship and harmony with nature.

**John:** It's been an interesting journey. I would suggest that once, in some form, we were not separated from a state of unity. In the time of early humans, before the so-called modern era, I believe many tribes, or groups of people, had a rich and deep connection with nature. However, as the human mind developed, we became separated. Part of that development is an expansion, which we term colonisation. Colonisation destroys cultures and nature, and also spreads or disseminates culture around the globe; it certainly spreads plants globally. In our industrialised or technologically developed society, it seems we have focused more on the organisation of society; to the extent there are large masses of people concentrated in certain areas, with little or no contact with the nature of the Earth that supports them, and at the same time, requiring huge resources to support their lifestyles and survival.

There's enormous separation in that! How do we get back into harmony with our intrinsic nature and the nature energy of the Earth we live on? The changes in climate around the globe will ensure that. In some ways, we have become so comfortable in our human-focused condition, the only way to wake up and find what is real and appropriate for the combined harmony of Earth and beings, is through radical change in ways of living, and in consciousness.

A catalyst for radical change is to come into stillness of mind, as opposed to constant busyness. In stillness we can discover the essence of self and our own nature, and the basic laws of healing and well-being. It is imperative we discover this.

**Rose:** You're saying the most important thing is being still?

## Connecting with Higher Mind

**John:** Yes, stillness of mind also enables us to access what is known as Higher Mind. This is a place of mind not separated, but connected to a more universal state of mind, an innate wisdom. You could call it God wisdom, a wisdom of truth and harmony, wherein lies respect and love for all. In separation, which appears to be the human state, there is a me-and-you state of mind, instead of thinking of us all together. Yet we are moving towards that place of togetherness. Again, I think stillness of mind leads us there, because we can see in stillness and quietness, our sense of unity.

**Rose:** Pulling the threads together, I've gathered that one of your passions is yoga, other passions are esoteric study, working with the body, and working with nature. All these are connected, and have a common focus on being really present, observing, and being with what is.

**John:** I sometimes feel I'm just beginning. I have all these different threads I'm working with. I really enjoy them, because they involve working with people and working with the nature of the Earth and plants; perhaps in some way bringing the two together. Then there's the deeper aspect, where I work with groups on a subjective or meditative level. In a sense, we are aiming to work with the focused will of God, bringing God's will or the basic natural laws into being. To do that, we have to move aside from the individual will, or maybe use that will to make sure it contacts the Highest-Vibration-That-Is, for the good of all. This is going on throughout the world on the human plane and beyond. If we look at the concept of fractals we can see how each small part represents some greater whole. At my best, I can hold the thought of connectedness to a universal energy or truth, and bring it into whatever work I am doing. In the end, it is not what I do, but what I convey through my being, which is of service to wholeness and unity.

## *Becoming more conscious is a commitment to a process of deepening self discovery*

The process of deepening consciousness can be both thrilling and very demanding. It requires a certain kind of vigilance; a willingness to face, embrace and take responsibility for aspects of self we do not like; the courage to feel the pain of being human and incomplete, and to move through our fear to greater wholeness. Sometimes, we are called to release old patterns or self images, with which we have become so identified, we're not even sure we can survive without them. Yet we not only survive but expand through this letting go.

This deep delving process of becoming more conscious involves a more intimate relationship with death, so we may live more fully. Death comes in many forms: ongoing surrender of the ego or "little self"; the collapse of old ways and loss of certainty; the courage to face clear-eyed the extinction of so many species on our planet; the killing of so many of our own species by war and predation; the sickness and dying of friends and family as a result of toxic emotions, stress, or environmental pollutants. Each time death shows up the challenge arises: how much do I really want to live? What is keeping me from a fully lived, passionate life? What can I do right now to express my aliveness?

# *Shift Seven*

## From self interest and exploitation to choosing to live in harmony.

With the realization of the essential interconnectedness of all life comes a responsibility to be of service to our interconnection. Living our passion as Love-in-action, we choose to exercise our creative freedom most fully through taking responsibility. Thus we become participants and co-creators in a creative universe.

# Mirjam Busch and Rudolf Jarosewitsch
## Spaciousness and the challenge of differentiation in conscious relationship.

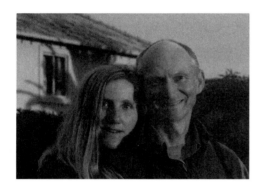

Mirjam Busch and Rudolf Jarosewitsch have been living a conscious partnership and working separately and together as counsellors/psychotherapists (MNZAC) with individuals, couples and groups for the last ten years. They started their relationship with a conscious choice and clear intention to follow a soul journey of discovery and growth. It is a vibrant relationship due to their willingness to stay open to the unexpected and to embrace challenges that present themselves. Both treasure the support of good friends and chosen family who give them a sense of belonging in their country of choice, New Zealand. Their vision is to live in a conscious community on the land in close connection to nature. www.partnering.inet.net.nz

**Mirjam:** There's a spaciousness that comes with the clarity of completely saying "no" to everything I don't want to do any longer. It creates a very new dimension. It's amazing! It opens up this huge, vast emptiness. I have this clarity, yet I really have a profound not knowing what's going to happen next!

**Rose:** Is it an empty creative space?

**Mirjam:** It's a very empty creative space because I'm really giving myself permission to say no. I'm closing doors and allowing myself to enter back into my own spaciousness, really. It's a strange sense;

I'm still grieving the past, but in the present I feel very clear, with this profound sense of not knowing.

**Rose:** Is there excitement in it?

**Mirjam:** I haven't quite touched the excitement. It's still more a sense of bewilderment. My inner child can't believe I've actually done what I've done. "Oh, my God, she really means it! She really will give us some space here. She really will listen!" The child is a bit stunned at my willingness to say, "Ok, right. I'm here."

**Rose:** You're going to take some time for you?

**Mirjam:** Absolutely! I'm just phasing out my clients slowly over the next month and then I'm really completely open to whatever emerges. I've never been in this place! This is a completely new place in my life! I've never ever given myself permission to go there!

**Rose:** It's a new adventure!

**Mirjam:** I don't know if it makes any sense to you?

**Rose:** Absolutely! I think it's a wonderful place to be. Particularly at this point in our collective history, to be able to be in a place of not knowing, is what we need to do. To be humble enough to say: "I don't know. I don't know the most important thing to do next." To let go of everything and just be!

**Mirjam:** Yes, to let go of all our patterns. I realize I've had a theme in my life of proving I'm good, so I will not be left. So I will be valued. Like a wandering adapted child. What's left when I let go of all that and everything associated with it? What will I be feeling? What will I be doing?

**Rose:** Who will you be?

**Mirjam:** I've no clue whatsoever!

**Rose:** You're willing to find out though?

**Mirjam:** It doesn't come from the will. The will can drag me into my patterns very easily. It's almost like my mind, body and heart have gone on strike. They won't participate any longer. I sit in supervision and I don't actually listen. My supervisor said, "It's going completely over your head, isn't it?" I said, "Yes. I'm not interested." I hear myself saying these things and think, "Oh, my God, what am I saying!" It is generally true I'm not interested any longer in pursuing my old adaptive patterns. My whole being cannot participate, so my mind shuts off. I don't even have a choice about it; it simply shuts off. I can't make myself adapt any longer. It's truly like something has gone on strike.

**Rose:** What you're saying fits perfectly into the exploration of consciousness in this book.

**Mirjam:** This is truly about consciousness and it's a new challenge for our relationship. We have to make room in our relationship to enter another dimension.

**Rose:** Are you and Rudolf going through this shift together?

*Shannon:*
*A Happiness Seed*

*I would nurture my WHOLE NEW WORLD seed. I would water it with love. I would blanket it with courteous soil. It would sprout from responsible fertilizer. As it would grow, it would grow into a world of eternal happiness without sin where everyone would not judge each other; they would look from the other person's point of view. Inside their heart is where the greatest things are lying. Seeds may be small, but with enough love and compassion they can grow into something magnificent. If I could sow a seed into a new world, my seed would have to be a happiness seed.*

**Mirjam:** Of course, Rudolf must be impacted by it because it's going to change our lives completely. We don't know how. He also has his own journey. He's getting to a stage where he'll probably have to confront his own patterns, and look at what he's really drawn to and interested in. We've no idea what this means to our relationship.

**Rose:** Did this process start in you?

**Mirjam:** It started in me. I'm usually the instigator of change in this relationship! It started in me about a year ago. I ignored it and denied it and felt challenged by it and tried to calm myself, convince myself, and stay focused. I almost numbed myself in order to manage life. Now it's become impossible to do that. My mind just won't go along with my old ways any longer. It just turns off and completely ignores my demands and my pushing. I sit there and my mind wanders off, forgets things, and drops things that aren't important. It says things I normally wouldn't say, rather truthfully so, and isn't concerned with appearing "as good". This feels inevitable. My mind is saying,"Ok, I'm going to take over now. I'm going to lead you, because if I don't, you're going to just stay with the familiar and with what you've learned."

**Rose:** It's your mind that's leading you?

**Mirjam:** I see my mind, in the Buddhist sense, as my heart. It's not a cognitive process. My mind and heart are very much connected and my mind works through my heart. It's actually protecting my heart. They're pairing up, and holding hands, and my mind's saying, "Right, somebody needs to look after your heart here."

**Rose:** Even though you're in the unknown, you feel safe?

**Mirjam:** I am safe, yet I've never been so profoundly in an unknown place. Inevitability is the best word. I don't have a choice about this. This is where I'm going. My job is just to surrender to it.

**Rose:** Do you find surrender easy?

**Mirjam:** Obviously, it hasn't been for forty-six years; because I didn't, but now I am. I'm simply noticing I am surrendering. I'm letting go of the gripping. I'm simply letting go and I don't know what evoked it or initiated it. It's been a slow awakening. I'm simply noticing that's what I do.

**Rose:** I imagine you have various tools and understandings that have prepared you to be able to surrender in this way and be in this place of not knowing without being afraid?

**Mirjam:** I think it was the experience of almost losing Rudolf when he was being operated on in open heart surgery. I was lying on the ground in the park, near the hospital. It was an incredible day, the sun was beaming, there was a deafening sound of cicadas all around me, and I lay on the grass spread eagled. I absolutely felt him in every tree, in every leaf. I totally felt myself merging with everything, including him. I knew exactly when the operation was over, to the minute! I knew also I was able to survive, whatever happened. I had to say goodbye to him before the operation. It was a very close encounter with death, with profound loss. It was an incredible experience, to find myself dissolving into the trees and feeling absolutely connected with him.

I had been overcome with terror at the thought of losing him and I went through, and past that. Now I've moved on to another journey, beyond terror or fear of loss.

**Rose:** Would you say your sense of self has changed since that moment?

**Mirjam:** Yes, I had a warm-up to profound loss and an experience of surviving that. I know now I have the ability to let go. Before, I didn't trust I knew how to do that. From there, it's been a slow letting go of friendships that aren't good for me. For example, suddenly realizing it's been a very one sided affair, years of being a good friend to somebody, who was not the least bit interested in my life. A real letting go. I just feel into myself and notice if I become drained when I'm with a person, situation, or conversation, and if I do, I let go. I'm doing a lot of shedding.

**Rose:** Would you say you are becoming more authentic?

**Mirjam:** I think so, but I'm not sure. It's so unfamiliar and I have no reference points for it. I don't even have a language for it. I'm entering a new world. So I really have to get to know the terrain. Who lives here? What language do they speak? What is the landscape like? What's the climate like? How does one live in this landscape? I don't know. I think I'm about to embark on the journey!

**Rose:** This all makes sense to me. Not that I know your experiences, but the process is familiar from my own experience, especially when you talk about the inevitability of it, and being in a new territory, and not knowing the language. I recognize that place of just being in the not knowing and surrendering.

**Mirjam:** What keeps coming to me is that it's a really profound "not knowing". There've been many times when I've not known what to do. This is a different "not knowing". This isn't a "not knowing" with the frustration of wanting an answer. It's really a "not knowing" without any need to have an answer! In the past, not knowing would make me restless. I'd go here, go there, see all these people to try and find an answer. I wanted them to tell me where I was, what I was meant to be doing, and where I was meant to be going. That's not what I want to do now.

**Rose:** This sounds a simpler place to be.

**Mirjam:** Yes. I'm just giving myself permission to really enter into the "not knowing" and not have to fix it or fill it with meaning and solutions. Instead of panicking and trying to make plans, "Oh God, where am I supposed to be? Who am I supposed to be with? "Trying to fill my life with purpose and meaning and direction, doesn't even work! Everything's becoming rather useless, and that's necessary, in order to enter into this spaciousness.

**Rose:** Is there any way you can relate what you're telling me to the idea of living your passion?

**Mirjam:** I think this is the seedbed. I really feel I'm preparing the ground! Completely and utterly preparing the conditions I need to, fully… I might be completely wrong, but if I let myself just speak… I imagine this may be really laying the ground for my true passion to flourish… this is preparing the soil.

**Rose:** Thank you. That makes sense as a possibility to me. Your image of the seedbed is perfect! Rudolf, I've been talking with Mirjam about where she is in her process and relating that to living her passion. Would you like to talk about what living your passion means to you?

**Rudolf:** To me, it has to do with conscious partnership and compassionate communication. I tie it into the challenge of differentiation. I think it's an ongoing challenge in every relationship: how to be your individual self and be in relationship? In the past, when Mirjam wanted to express herself, or do something that would scare me, I would, in a subtle way, put pressure on her. She put pressure on herself too, as her habitual pattern. I reinforced her pattern and she lost herself and wasn't aware how it happened. She's acutely aware now and she doesn't want to ever do that again.

**Rose:** She wanted to express something of herself that was threatening to you, and you would somehow subtly put pressure on her not to?

**Rudolf:** Yes, then she would give up her wish or her dream instead of exploring it.

**Rose:** I guess this affected the relationship in some negative way?

**Rudolf:** Yes, and the way I did it, I was coming from a place of fear, and this reinforced messages she had within herself.

**Rose:** Were you a mirror for her, so she could see her own fears and limiting beliefs?

**Rudolf:** Yes and when you're conscious, you can be aware of that. We weren't always conscious about this process. It just happened. Then you notice the energy or the caring has diminished. Living your passion means to be really vibrant, in the here and now, just present. Often, we slip into old familiar patterns and the love gets lost. My passion is to embrace the challenges that come in the relationship with Mirjam and to see whatever goes on for her is relevant to me too. One belief we've held in the work we've done with couples is not to separate out your issue and my issue, but to see they are somehow related to one another. My passion is to stay alive, stay on my feet, and embrace what's ahead of me. Mirjam is saying she's not happy. She needs some time out urgently. This makes absolute sense to me. I notice I've become stale in my work. I don't have the energy for it. On the other hand, there are thoughts about security, income, finances; all that doesn't allow me to look at my needs. I put up with it. What I very much appreciate about Mirjam is she's not willing to put up with it. When she feels something very acutely, she cannot ignore her truth.

**Rose:** Part of what I'm hearing you say is, for a relationship to stay vital, differences need to be expressed. Part of that is about expressing your own truth, which may be different from your partner's truth; and then you find a way to live with those differences?

**Rudolf:** Absolutely.

**Rose:** That's quite challenging, isn't it?

**Rudolf:** Yes, but I believe if we don't do that, there's a danger we fall into habitual patterns and routines. These might work for a while, but in the long run, they're detrimental. An indicator is, when the magic gets lost.

**Rose:** You're just going through the motions rather than being fully present?

**Rudolf:** That's right. Also, I noticed I would frequently try to prove something. That's a very undesirable condition. I like to be drawn to work rather than push myself. That's why I like the idea of taking a break. We talk about moving to the country and I think I could give the work away. Part of me likes the idea of planting a garden, working with the land. It's something I haven't done enough.

**Rose:** To get more down to earth?

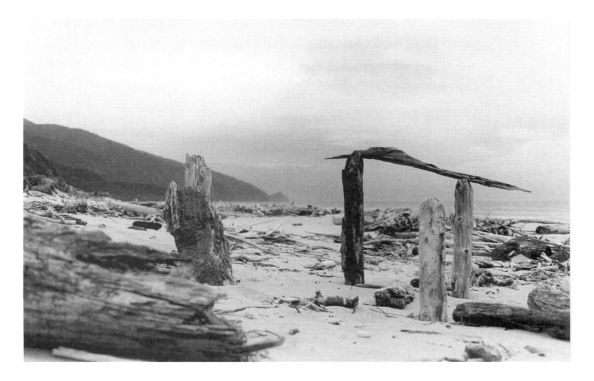

**Rudolf:** Yes, I've not always followed my passion in that way, been too much of a do-gooder, trying to do the right thing. This is what Mirjam reflected back to me, and I can recognize it in myself to some degree.

**Rose:** You made a distinction between your passion being drawn out, as opposed to pushing yourself to do something which results in feeling flat. It's interesting that the true meaning of education is to draw out.

**Rudolf:** What I've been wondering, and writing about, is my heart attack. From the readings I've done, I've found subtle stress is actually an indicator that leads to a heart attack. It's not the big stressful situations, but the subtle, ongoing chronic stress. I've been wondering how I've put myself under stress and discovering more and more of the subtleties of that, and trying to free myself from it.

**Rose:** There was an unaware stress to which you were so accustomed, you didn't even notice?

**Rudolf:** Exactly.

**Rose:** I also wonder about therapeutic work, which you've been doing for many years now, and if that puts a stress on the heart in some ways, because you're constantly responding to other people's pain and suffering.

**Rudolf:** Yes, after a while, there's something like compassion fatigue. You can no longer respond. Much as you want to, it becomes hard to empathise with another person. You've heard so many stories.

**Rose:** It sounds as though both of you have been in a pattern of pushing yourselves to be well adapted people and therapists, to be there for others and be helpful.

**Rudolf:** At the moment, talking with you, it feels like one of those turn-around places or crisis positions, where something new will happen. We both don't quite know what it will look like. The challenge is to be with the unknown, and I notice how often I either try to make plans or find another way to move out of it.

**Rose:** You don't feel so comfortable with being in the unknown?

**Rudolf:** I don't. Definitely not! That's when the habitual patterns come up again, such as wanting to force a decision. I keep remembering something said by a colleague, "Whenever I need to make a decision, I observe what I do." This pays tribute to the fact that decisions are whole body decisions, whereas a habitual pattern is to go into the head to try and figure something out, rather than just noticing what it is you do. I'd like to embrace that more. For instance, yesterday I was a bit tired and the Qi-Gong group was meeting. At first I thought I wouldn't go, then all of a sudden, I packed my things and went. That was something I noticed I just did rather than pushing myself to do it.

I think it's easier to live my passion when I observe what I do rather than when I put pressure on myself. A head decision comes more from old patterns of trying to please others, and that's the challenge I'm working with at the moment. It's Mirjam's challenge to me. I could have continued and had a second heart attack. When I really listen to what I want to do, part of me wants time to get back to the writing I've started about my heart. I call it, "Conversation with my heart".

**Rose:** Are there particular skills, tools, or understandings you've learned, to support you through working with differences. To find a way to be together in which you don't suppress yourselves or make yourselves less; so you can both be all you are? What have you learned about that?

**Rudolf:** What comes to mind are Virtue cards, from the Virtues Project. The Popovs looked at different world religions and discovered they have in common a number of virtues. These are the same in all the major religions: Christianity, Buddhism, Hinduism, Judaism, and so on. They themselves are Baha'I, and they believe in the unity of all religions, so they founded the Virtues Project and compiled a list of virtues. We've done a course with them and attend a regular "Virtues Group" once a month, where the focus is on one particular virtue. It's uplifting to talk about something positive. Mirjam and I have a set of cards, each day we pull a card and sometimes we share this with each other.

**Mirjam**: They've been helpful when we're self righteously stuck in our own patterns and unable to see a way through. I remember being really, really stuck on the way to a holiday together. I was furious with Rudolf and thought he needed to be more considerate. Well, which card did he pick? Consideration! Then I thought, "Well right! This is exactly what you need!" Which card did I pick? Consideration! And we actually picked these cards four days in a row, out of fifty-two cards! By then, we were both humbled enough to really ponder what consideration means! The cards give you not only the quality of the virtue, but also the actions. I think often, when we're stuck, we simply don't have the wisdom to know what's appropriate, and we need some guidance. We let ourselves be guided by these cards, which reflect human qualities we all carry. They are a good reminder of what we already have and this is helpful, because I think we can lose the plot many times in a relationship!

**Rose:** There's the mirror again! In the work Woods and I have been doing together around becoming more conscious in relationship, the ways we mirror each other have become very apparent. Whenever I react to something in his behaviour, it turns out to be exactly what I'm doing! I can't see it in myself, but I can see it in him! Sometimes the accuracy of the mirroring feels quite uncanny, and it reminds me how I need relationship in order to see those parts of myself I'm otherwise blind to.

**Mirjam:** That's right! It's very clear in the other person! There is an equality going on. Another tool for us has been the understanding; we're equally wounded but also equally capable. We don't have an imbalance where we think one of us is more or less than the other: more wounded, more capable, more spiritually advanced, or anything. We simply respect the fact we've come together because we're equal.

**Rose:** Has that always been present in your relationship?

**Rudolf:** I think when you've come together, as we have, on a soul journey, there's a clear indication it's a learning relationship. That's why difficulties or conflicts are always learning opportunities. We both choose to embrace those rather than to shy away from them.

**Mirjam:** It was a huge, huge shift for us when we actually consciously chose to see difficulties as opportunities, not as evidence we're incompatible. They're actually an invitation for us to grow, and that means we don't see difficulties as threats, we see them truly as stepping stones.

**Rose:** Does that mean you don't take offence when differences emerge between you?

**Mirjam:** We may temporarily, but I think it's supported our ability to let the problem work and to hang in with each other. I don't think we could have hung in otherwise. We would simply have given up, if we hadn't seen difficulties as opportunities for mutual and spiritual growth. This means, as much as we might react to these difficulties, and all our patterns flare up, and we say or do all sorts of unhelpful things to each other, there is still an underlying strong belief, or faith, we need to hang in, in order to find out what the gift is. It gives us the discipline, perseverance, and resilience to stay committed to working through our difficulties. We often look back from a stronger, more peaceful place, and are relieved we persevered to reap the rewards.

**Rose:** This is in the context of understanding your relationship as a soul relationship?

**Mirjam:** In the beginning we asked what we wanted from one another and it was very clear this was going to be a healing relationship.

**Rose:** You both wanted that, and chose each other because of that?

**Mirjam:** Yes, we knew this was about a healing journey, which means we can only heal if our wounds have permission to come to the surface.

**Rose:** It's challenging, isn't it, for one to stay present and loving when the other is reacting from a wounded part of self? How long have you been together now?

**Rudolf:** Ten years.

**Rose:** Do you find the work of relationship keeps going on and on?

**Mirjam:** Yes, it changes, and goes deeper, and then it changes again. Whenever we get to a place where one of us is saying, usually me, "I think we need to separate", it usually means we need to separate from the old relationship we've had, and build a new relationship. So it's not so much the need to physically separate, as much as the need to enter into a new phase of relationship with each other.

**Rose:** Somehow, you find inside yourselves, the commitment to keep going to the next level?

**Rudolf:** When difficulties arise through very habitual responses, when I want to change Mirjam and say, "If only she were different", I believe this is a mild form of violence. The nonviolent approach would be to see I'm part of the equation and ask the question: in what way is this part of me? What is the part of me I don't like? This is both very empowering to me and respectful to her.

**Rose:** I was listening last night to a cd by Marshall Rosenberg, called "*Speaking Peace*", and I've read his book, "*Nonviolent Communication*". I find his approach is founded on some very sound values and principles and I believe you've been working with these?

**Rudolf:** I think it's important in a relationship to read together, to continue learning. Rosenberg's was one of the books we read together. In his approach, difficulties arise as an expression of an unmet need or a discounted feeling. So to ask the questions: what do I feel? And what do I need? And to take time to tune in and find the answers is a very useful tool. Rather than getting stuck, or becoming reactive, I learn to be more reflective. We also spend lots of time sitting in a spa pool. We're both water signs, so water seems to have some healing qualities for us, just sitting in a spa together, letting things flow.

**Mirjam:** Thinking about difference, what's hard for me, is to endure the little differences in our personalities and the way we do things, which can be so grating and irritating. It's not the big things usually, it's the day to day little things that really frustrate and irritate me the most. I think we need to embrace our limits and be really honest and truthful about saying, "I don't want to live with that any longer." Rather than make ourselves endure something that really impacts our well-being. On the other hand, we could also learn to play with difference, and sometimes we do this very well.

**Rose:** What if the other person isn't able to change the thing which is so irritating?

**Mirjam:** Often they can't, or won't, because it's so much a part of who they are! We need to know those parts of the other person we don't want to live with, and arrange our living situations accordingly. We don't want to end up making a contract to endure each other at all costs. That kills joy and love in a relationship.

**Rudolf:** I can always change myself, hard as it may be at times. As I do so, the relationship changes. For me, it's worth hanging in; as long as I can embrace there is something for me to learn. Discomfort and pain are usually not welcome, but an urgent reminder an old habit is no longer useful. A helpful question for me has been, "What is being asked of me in this situation I am not happy with?"

**Rose:** It's very delicate, isn't it? As we've been going down through the layers working consciously with relationship, Woods and I have recognized the reactivity that surfaces in relationship is common to the human condition and is not to be taken too personally. That's why it's such important work to do. If relatively conscious people find it so difficult to live together, and you multiply that into the world, that's where wars stem from! It's all a continuum of how difficult it is to live with differences. That's what I remind myself when I'm running out of patience, "Oh, my goodness, this is vital work!" *Laughter.*

**Mirjam:** Absolutely. We do this for humanity, not only for ourselves. As well, relationships help to pull me out of self absorption.

**Rose:** Thank you for your intimate interview about being in the space of not knowing, and sharing so much about your highly conscious relationship.

## *We are spiritual beings and spirit is unlimited*

Shifting our focus from "having what we want" to BEING WHO WE DEEPLY ARE will create a more peaceful way forward for humanity. We *are* spiritual beings having a human experience. Each of us carries a spark of the Divine and has the potential to unfold the creative process consciously. We *can* discover and invent new and more ingenious ways of living together on this beautiful planet Earth; ways in which we can share life's natural abundance, everyone has enough, and our relationships with each other, and with nature, are sacred. The people in this book believe this is what we are called to do at this time of global transformation: to connect with our essential nature; to live in service to our highest visions for humanity and life on Earth; to be Love-in-action.

# *Shift Eight*

## A shift in identity occurs when we recognize we are not our thoughts and commit to mastering our minds.

The realization there is intelligence beyond individual mind, more powerful than thought, awakens us to a new dimension of consciousness and the recognition we are not who we thought we were. We may then choose to develop a discipline which supports us to withdraw our attention from negative thinking and limiting belief patterns in order to focus attention on our creative powers.

# Jonathan Evatt
## Writing at the borderland

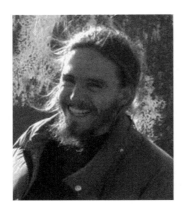

Jonathan's purpose at this time is to share and explore the timeless Path of Freedom (a Path with a Heart) with those interested in setting themselves free from the confusion and suffering so typical in the world today. He is presently writing a series of books sharing a body of wisdom at once deeply pragmatic, down-to-earth, and spiritually profound in its ramifications. His approach to spirituality, Life, and living is an integral one that draws people's attention toward the essential empowerment of who and what they are in this moment, rather than pursuing some lofty ideal of what is possible in a never eventuating future. His personal website is at www.jonathanevatt.com

**Jonathan**: Living my passion comes back to a choiceless choice: ultimately that's all I can do, although I may appear to choose otherwise. The word "passion" has its origins with the Passion of the Christ, which referred to his suffering and his trial and tribulation, battling with what he had to go through. Certainly for me, the Universe is always presenting me with a challenge as it manifests through me from moment to moment. One can suffer that challenge or simply approach it wisely and derive from it whatever's to be derived. From the perspective I come from, whether you win a million dollars or lose a million dollars, it's a challenge! It's only the ego mind that turns around and says one's a good thing and one's a bad thing and I want one and not the other. Whereas for the Presence that is, they're neither good nor bad and the resulting triumph within that challenge is a greater embodiment of one's power.

Living my passion is about remaining present with the challenge that's forever presenting itself in many different forms.

**Rose:** Are you saying it's all a challenge?

**Jonathan:** I think reality itself is a challenge. There's universal power challenging personal power to come forth, to come into body, into carnation, into the flesh. That's just an innate part of this human realm.

**Rose:** It's interesting you refer to the Passion of the Christ because I always think of the Crucifixion as a metaphor for the crucifixion of the ego on the cross of soul. As we're challenged to evolve, our attachment to ego identification inevitably brings suffering. Or, another way of putting it is, at times the human in us is in painful conflict with our spiritual destiny.

**Jonathan**: In my approach to life and the path one takes, I don't relate so much to the idea it is this thing called "ego" that is bad, which one somehow has to get around or overcome. The origin of the word ego is Latin for "I". It's possible in the physical world; we are the only animal to develop that; the only physical life form to take on a felt sense of the "I". It's not so much that the ego has to be gotten rid of or transcended. The sense of self arising through the "I", or ego self, is based on an identity derived from the exterior, rather than the interior. That's not a bad thing. It's just part of the evolution of things, of the stage life is going through. We can look at some of the destructive tendencies the ego-self has and conclude ego is a bad thing: look at all this pain it's creating! I don't even see the ego as something that exists; it's just a misidentification of what I am. If I start thinking I'm this candle here on this table, well that's going to create certain difficulties, especially if you lean over and blow it out! Likewise, if I start thinking I'm this body, this body is me, this is what I am, that also has some inherent challenges or problems. The human collective, and every individual within it, has to face the challenge of what we identify with. Perception shifts through facing this challenge and great *power* results from this.

## The Challenge of becoming more inclusive

**Rose:** Are you saying the challenge is in bringing forth our own power by withdrawing our identification with the ego-self?

**Jonathan:** Ultimately what we're being challenged to do is shift our perception to one which is increasingly more inclusive. The perception of the ego-self in most men and women is fairly exclusive. It cuts out a lot of what is there and tends to stick to some fairly ingrained beliefs about what is and what isn't. Certainly for the last little while, we've been stuck in this whole superstition of materialism. Well, not so much stuck in it as going through the challenge of it, and the challenge we're facing is to become more inclusive.

How do I keep expanding my perception to include more of what is? To include the ego, but also to include more of what "I" really is? Initially we start out thinking the "I" is my body and my history: born on this date to these parents, and all the rest of it. However one can expand that perception to a point where there's the realization the "I" that I am, is the "I" that you are, which is also the "I" we call God. And it's all the same! It's still ego according to the roots of that word. It's still I. Ultimately, this "I" is much more expanded; now it includes everything. The experience arising within this expanded sense of "I" is the sense of *self* or "I" disappearing. What is *self* when there is no longer some-*thing* we can identify as *non-self*?

**Rose:** Instead of there being an "I" and many "its", in reality, there is no separation? Everything is part of One Presence? How does this relate to living your passion, Jonathan?

**Jonathan:** I find I get moved and excited about certain things. One is the writing I'm doing. I guess living one's passion is staying present to that excitement, the sense of compulsion to do and explore certain things. Some of the things we're talking about, and I'm writing about, are the evolving result of simply following what feels true and real to me; which in my case, and again if we come back to the original meaning of the word passion, has at times been something I've had to endure. I think mainly because, as a youth I didn't understand what I felt passionate about, or interested in, was way out of the scope of what most people around me seemed to even be aware of, let alone interested in, and if I talked to them, they wouldn't even know what I was going on about.

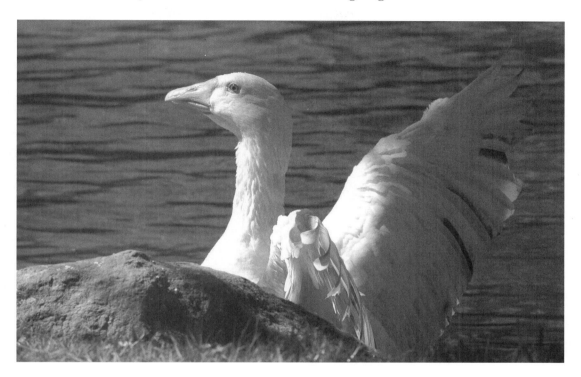

## A choiceless choice

**Rose:** This exploration is something you've been engaged in since your youth?

**Jonathan:** Again that's why I'd say it's a choiceless choice. At the human level, I don't really feel I have much of a say in the matter; it was just pushing its way through me. It just had to happen. The human element of me certainly may have been under the illusion it had some choice about what was happening. My sense, in hindsight, is really all I was getting to choose, if there was any choice at all, was how painful I was going to make it. If I choose to do something other than what is flowing through from the spiritual side of me, things start to get painful, complicated and difficult.

**Rose:** If you resist?

**Jonathan**: Yeah, like a little resistor on an electrical circuit; it starts to heat up and it can heat up so much it burns out. Whereas, if we take that little resistor out of the line, suddenly there's much more charge pumping through to the other end of the wire and you can do something with it. It's useful. It seemed I had choices to either resist or not resist, but the pain would soon get me to realize, well, what am I doing? Perhaps I need to change my approach to things.

**Rose:** As a youth did you feel quite isolated?

**Jonathan:** I did, socially. Having said that, there was some other level where I didn't feel isolated, because I always felt connected to some-*thing*. There was always some-*thing* much bigger than my limited sense of me, or "I". In that sense, I guess the play on words I've taken from it all is, we're all ultimately alone, and that word itself means All-One. When I come into All-One-ness, I stand alone. There's only one "I", yet it doesn't have to be a lonely affair. To me, loneliness is a social phenomenon, when it happens; whereas, All-One-ness is a state that's always there, whether we're tuned into it or not. At times I've felt socially apart from things, but then I'm aware I also made it that way. There was part of me that really didn't want to be part of things. I was quite defensive about sociality and the culture around me coming in too much. I'd just be slightly dismayed at anything socially 'in' - this is the kind of sunglasses to have - my whole being wouldn't want to go near it. I've never been a tea or coffee drinker for that reason, because everyone seemed to do it, sort of compulsively.

**Rose:** In terms of sociality, I know for me it's been a journey to find words for the experiences I've had. The more I'm able to find words, the more I'm able to connect with others and with my experience, rather than having to disconnect from one or the other.

**Jonathan:** Experience is actually coming out of the unknown, so there's no way to put it into words. Certainly the known I inherited from my culture didn't incorporate much of that stuff, and here it is bursting its way out of the unknown! People like you, and others, feel that occurring. You can't put it into words until it gets integrated and then it can be described in some way. It becomes part of one's 'known'. I look at that 'known' as information, and in-formation is bringing into form. As 'stuff' comes out of the unknown, we gather the in-formation pertaining to it and thus map out the unknown into our 'known'.

**Rose:** That's why I write: to bring stuff through from the unknown to the known. Is it the same for you too?

**Jonathan:** As far as the writing goes? Yes, when I get out of the way of it all. *Laughter.*

**Rose:** Do you enjoy writing?

**Jonathan:** I do. Sometimes I'll exert too much effort at a human level, if I can use that term, to do the writing, but then the end result won't feel right. So when it comes to revising, I'll end up stripping stuff out or changing it a lot. I find much of what comes up in the writing comes when I'm approaching the reality around me. I'm having a conversation with someone, or watching a movie, or even reading a book; that's already a big thing full of information. Just as I am with that, the unknown is also there. So here's this known thing - a book or a movie or whatever - the unknown is permeating through it, and I'll gain a whole lot of information that wasn't necessarily there. I'll walk out of that room, or flick through a few pages of the book, and suddenly there's a vast amount of knowledge I can really feel in the body that came from somewhere. It wasn't from the book because it didn't appear from those pages, but it was through reading those pages my attention was taken in a particular direction.

**Rose:** So where is the information coming from? Is there's some sort of information-laden energy that you are a vehicle for, or you're putting yourself in service to?

**Jonathan:** My sense is, at the most profound level, it's all One Thing. It's not as if there's even this human self as a separate entity. It may be experienced that way from the perspective of the rational mind, but the way I see it is, it's all one vast field of intelligence, of Life manifesting as the form of life, which is what we call the world. Life is much vaster and more ineffable than the form side of life. This thing we are, this "I", is also Life. None of it really comes from anywhere. It's all just arising. I'm glad you didn't use the word channeling, the whole notion of which I've never understood. It's always seemed very dualistic to me. Here I am this self, very separate from everything, and here's this other entity somewhere floating around out in the ether and relaying all this information to this "me" and then I'm sending it out to the world. It seems very segmented.

**Rose:** I agree. Words can be very inaccurate, so anything I say is a kind of fumbling around to find ways to communicate with you. I do have the sense that there's a noosphere, or field of consciousness, and some of us are tuned in to that at a certain level of consciousness. We're all thinking within the same field and interpreting it in our own way, through our own particular preferred ways of expressing our passion. There's some energy we're expressing, which we're part of, and participating in. I feel, at my best moments, I'm living on an unfolding edge of consciousness, and the people I'm connected with, we're all sort of dancing on this edge, and not so much understanding it, as extending it. Whatever it is, is happening and unfolding through us. What I think I'm hearing you say, is that your passion is to be in that?

## The borderland between the known and the unknown

**Jonathan:** Well that's where all the action is! *Laughter.* That edge you talk about, I experience as the borderland between the known and the unknown, and our challenge is to be constantly incorporating, through a shift in perception, more of the unknown into the known. A lot of people, I think, shy away from that edge and become fixed on the known. The unknown does try to present itself; it always will. Rather than facing the challenge as a challenge from the unknown, we'll perceive it as a problem with the known because that's where our attention is fixated. Oh God, now the known's breaking down! We need to adjust the known to fix this thing and get rid of it. There are lots of examples we could use, maybe someone loses his job, his wife leaves him, he nearly dies in a car crash, and it looks like his whole life has nearly gone down the chute. Most people interpret this as "something's gone wrong with my known" and start asking, "How do I adjust my known and get it back to the way that feels comfortable?" As opposed to embracing whatever it is that's coming from the unknown.

It's being on that edge again. It's an intense place to be. I see the connection between intention and in tension. It's only on that border-land between the known and the unknown, I start to feel the intention of the isness flowing through this whole experience. Being there in that intention, I also go into tension. The word tension relates to a condition of being stretched. In this case, it's my perception and awareness being stretched. It's a very tense, alive sort of place to be. It's quite fiery, yet at the same time; it's also very soft, silent and still. For the ego-self, that also can be quite intense, like the discomfort most people feel when they're with someone and there's absolute silence, sitting in a car without talking, for instance. There's something uneasy about that. My sense is silence takes the person closer to the edge of the unknown, because if we're sitting here in silence, there's much less of the known to engage with. I'll start to get into the unknown! Maybe I'll feel what that person's feeling, or I'll sense the history of the car, or whatever. That's usually too much for the ego-self, so most people pull back to the known and start talking.

**Rose:** You could say this is what's happening globally as well. The known appears to be breaking down and there are lots of different ways to interpret this. We could see it as disaster, or we could live on the edge and be excited by the new.

**Jonathan:** I think really we're being faced with an incredible opportunity for massive collective growth. You're absolutely right. Everywhere things are breaking down. Political and environmental systems are breaking down. Financial systems are all held together by nothingness, because all the money's actually been stripped out by a few greedy people who think they need it all. All that stuff constitutes the known, and it's getting pretty fragile. That really does present humanity, or that aspect of Life manifesting as this thing we call humanity, with an amazing opportunity to make some very large leaps in perception. I sometimes wonder if it was necessary to do it all in such a large leap, or could we have just incrementally adjusted as we went along? If people were living in a way that was conscious of reality, of how things operate, could we have made that progression over a longer period of time? For whatever reason, certainly looking at the history of any organism, things do seem to happen in these huge leaps, far more so than we ever realize. For example, some archeologists claim mountain ranges like the Andes and the Rockies running down through America were formed in a couple of days. There are stories, people who used to live there at the time, were an ocean going people, and literally overnight their land was elevated by five to six thousand feet! Those who survived had to deal with a whole different reality.

**Rose:** We seem to be a species which has pushed itself right to an edge and this is causing us to leap in order to survive. This seems to me to be connected with the suffering aspect of passion you were talking about earlier. From the suffering, or from the tension of living one's passion on the edge, comes the motivation for the leap. Maybe if there wasn't that edge or that tension or that suffering, we would just all hang out! *Laughter.* Why would we bother to do anything?

## *We all need a mirror*

**Jonathan:** There's a body of knowledge called Huna, which was very prevalent in Hawaii, and indeed still practiced. It has been said, for something like 1600 years, there was a very enlightened society of people who lived by the principles of Huna. According to Huna history, there was no crime and no murder, for example, in stark contrast to today's society. They had no army, no police, or any laws at all! It was a particular cosmology of reality and life that seemed to work at the time. One of the core principles in Huna is: everyone is a divine being. And as a divine being, there is only one need: a need for a mirror. In my reality, this thing we call the world is that mirror. The degree to which I forget my true nature as a divine being and the degree to which I start thinking I'm something else, is the degree to which I will start making life-taking choices. In Huna, there's no right and wrong. There's no good and bad. There's simply that which is life-giving and that which is life-taking. If I make life-taking choices, the consequences will be painful to experience. It's perfect, because pain gives us the signal: "Oh, Ok, I'm making a life-taking choice." Or, "I'm approaching reality in a way that's life-taking. What is it I'm forgetting about myself?" According to these principles, certainly pain is very much a key element. I think at a certain point in our development as human beings, we get to a stage where we don't have to experience pain. The moment I become aware I'm not feeling at peace, becomes my threshold now, "Oh, I don't feel at peace right now. What am I forgetting about my true nature?" Whereas some people literally have to obliterate their physical body and die physically, and go through that pain in order to review their situation. The spirit welling within will, in a moment of extraordinary pain, realize something; remember something, like a jolt to the system. Hopefully we're moving on, sooner rather than later, to a place where it doesn't have to be so painful.

**Rose:** Do you think the core aim is to remember our divinity?

**Jonathan:** Yes. We are mysterious, magical beings which we've only just started to fathom, and over time, we will awaken to our magnificence.

**Rose:** Do you have any sense of mission to teach this to other people?

**Jonathan**: The human side of me would see it that way, but to integrate that back into my approach to things: yes, there is this sense of sharing. On the one hand, within the realm of dualistic reality we live in, yeah I know something, I've learned something, and I'm going to teach and impart that to other people, so they might experience it. The reality I experience behind all that is actually, that's not what's happening at all, because within the totality of things, I can't even put it into words!

One day I was sitting in a ten day meditation retreat in Switzerland and we were asked to contemplate what it would mean if we were no longer waiting. It was an exercise we were given to do. For some reason, that was the perfect thing to do in that moment! It was just the trigger, and I went through this whole succession of thoughts penetrating from the most basic level to the most profound. And suddenly, pumpf, I just didn't exist anymore! There was just awareness! I don't know how long I was in just awareness, because there wasn't any time anymore. At some point I was able to gain use of my thinking mind again, "Well, what's going to move me? There's nothing to do. Everything's perfect. Everything! Everyone and everything that's happening, it's all perfect, so why am I going to get up from here? If I did, what would I bother doing? There's nothing to do!" And I thought: "Well, why did the Buddha get up and why did he do what he did for sixty something years?" There was an innate sense this was a state enlightened beings tapped into, so what moved them?

Then what came to me was an image of a hand. Here were these fingers and they were all kind of arthritic. Suddenly the thumb for some reason was able to move. It reconnected with the wholeness of the body. The body is the totality; what we could call God. The thumb was moving and there was a sense the whole body was going to create a compulsion for that thumb to start pushing on the other fingers, to wake them up, or to move them. They've been arthritic for so long they don't know they can move. They think this rigidity they're experiencing is just the way it is. The thumb is going to start pushing the finger this way and that, and as that finger starts experiencing different positions, it realizes, "Oh, I can move!" And then it will keep experiencing movement to a greater and greater degree. The thumb might have the illusion it was running around separate from these fingers and doing something to them. However, in reality, the totality now is ripe to move. Does that make sense? I find it hard to put these things into words.

**Rose:** I think so. You seem to be talking about how movement happens within the collective. We are all one interconnected field of consciousness, so when one person wakes up, the ripples of that awakened energy inevitably starts to affect others, to move them, and the movement spreads. Like you, I've had a sense at times; I really didn't have to do anything. Just receiving information was enough to bring it more into the collective consciousness. I didn't even have to write. I didn't have to do anything! All I had to do was be conscious. Then there'd be another moment, and I'd start to put language to the experience, communicating and interacting again. The whole process had a feeling of being a choiceless choice. Do you sense what you're doing is contributing something of value to humanity at this time, and does that matter to you?

**Jonathan:** I would only be guessing because I think at the end of the day, what constitutes *value* very much depends on who's deriving the value. I'll only really know that when the material is out there, and these fingers, so to speak, that are all over the place, come back and tell me they have derived value from it. Then I can see something has shifted that was life-giving within the world of those people. Certainly I've already had some feedback to that effect, but as I'm writing, I don't have the sense I'm doing this for any reason. It just sort of has to happen. It just is there. Just as, suddenly you get the urge to pee you've just got to go and have a pee. You don't make a big deal out of it, and God only knows what that pee's going to do as it goes through the water systems of the entire planet, which ultimately are going to have some atom of that pee in them. I don't have to think about all that. I just have the urge to do something. So I'm doing it!

## *When we link heart to heart and mind to mind, we create One World*

There is a global network of conscious change makers linking up like the imaginal cells which carry the new genetic code in the metamorphosis of chrysalis to butterfly. At first, the chrysalis sensing the new cells are foreign, kills them, but as the new cells proliferate, the chrysalis gives up. Then the imaginal cells can use the substance of the outgoing form of the chrysalis to create the new, freer form of the butterfly.

What if the social innovations being created now are the imaginal cells carrying the DNA for a new world? As the new consciousness begins to resonate through us, all around the world we are waking up to our capacities to be conscious change makers, and to the power of our interconnectedness. Linking both through the Internet and through the power of intentional thought and meditative consciousness, as in the recent global meditation, Fire the Grid, we are starting to sense the possibility our collective thoughts and heart-felt energy, may be enough to shift consciousness on the planet, and allow a new story for humanity to emerge.

# Anahata and Orah Ishaya
## 64,000 enlightened individuals could transform the whole planet.

**Anahata Ishaya**: Nee: July 25, 1952, Quebec City, Quebec, Canada. Extraordinary life moments include wonderful and loving parents, three great siblings and their families, two beautiful children, a phenomenal extended family, two enlightening ex-husbands, an angelic host of incredible friends, kind and giving neighbours, many caring teachers, numerous supportive 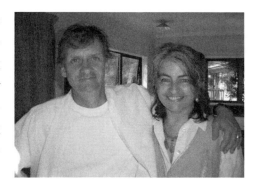 employers, six special staff, the Earthly love of my life, Orah, four unconditionally loving Avatars, and all with the Grace of the One. Presently present: Nelson, New Zealand.

**Orah Ishaya**: I am a Dutch-born New Zealander and the second of four sons. During my youth, sport was the focus of my life and school something to be endured. The sport led to a career in physical education; the school made it a short career. I retrained in physiotherapy, the occupation I have worked in since. In tandem with career, there has been family; I have two grown sons. As the interest in spirituality grew, physiotherapy became a vehicle to realize who I am, and is an expression of that interest. I am grateful to all my friends for helping me to see the various persons called Orah. It is to the love of my life, Anahata, I am most grateful. She keeps pointing the way back to my own heart. There is unlimited gratitude to Sri AmmaBhagavan for giving me the experience of divinity, which means I argue less with life and experience much more Joy!!

Some ten years ago, I received a phone call, out of the blue, asking me if I'd like to help organize a workshop for the Ishaya's Ascension in Nelson. I had no idea how this person knew my name but, as I listened, something caught my attention, and I said yes. That began a three year involvement for me with Ascension and hosting Ascension teachers in my home. Different teachers came each time, travelling to New Zealand from the Centre for the Society for Ascension, (SFA) in North Carolina, USA. I deeply admired their commitment to their spiritual path. They were thoroughly modern lay people, living as wandering monks and teachers, then returning to SFA for periods of intense meditation and group processing. The practice of Ascension focuses around ancient words of wisdom which charm the mind and develop attitudes of praise, gratitude, love and compassion. I found it a very helpful practice which gave me greater peace, clarity, and detachment. I didn't meet Anahata and Orah until later, when we were sitting in satsang with another spiritual teacher, Maitreya. They talk here about their spiritual quests, which led them to become teachers of Ascension, and about Anahata's experience of being with MSI, the enlightened Master and founder of SFA, who left his body in 1997. More recently, Anahata and Orah became givers of Deeksha, or the Oneness Blessing, a powerful spiritual transmission.

**Anahata:** I always considered my life to be full of passion even though it wasn't always fulfilled. I wanted to be a clothing designer from the time I was very young, about six or seven years old; it was very instilled in me. At nine years old, I was sewing my own clothes, making patterns and sewing for other people. I didn't get clothes off the rack until much later in life, and by the time I was, let's say about seventeen, there was nowhere I could go to college for clothes designing in Canada. So the passion part of that went out the window rather depressively. That first passion never left me but it was replaced with a different kind of passion. It was much later, when I turned thirty eight, when the passion of getting to know God really came to me in full force. I heard my girlfriend say: "Well, you know we're all One, don't you?" This totally changed my life.

**Rose:** Just like that?

**Anahata**: Just like that! This one sentence took me out of one world and shifted me into another. All of a sudden, my brain, heart and being went: "What is this? What's this all about? I have to know!" From then on, it was a continuous search for that Oneness.

**Rose:** Sounds very dramatic. You saw the light!

**Anahata**: I guess, even though I didn't know it was a light at the time. I do feel I had no choice in my life after that. It became my beacon and I followed it like a moth to a flame. There were many detours, but the major thrust of it was to know, to find out what it meant, that we are all One.

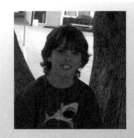

*Callum:*
*An Expanding Seed*

My WHOLE NEW WORLD seed is a speck of pollen from a buttercup. It will grow into a huge tree with a magnificent height of five hundred metres. The vines on the tree will give off a strange gas containing peace, strength and courage every twelve hours. The trees roots will also grow fifty metres every half hour, expanding the world at the same rate so everyone can stay on the world forever and still live in comfort.

**Rose:** I know you've both dedicated yourselves to your spiritual paths, through your work as teachers of Ascension and as Deeksha givers.

**Anahata**: Yes, it became the main ingredient in my life. Also, when it came to our relationship, we put that, our common vision, first. It happened naturally. Anything we did, or that happened between us, or how we communicated, we knew was to help us get clearer in that ultimate goal.

**Rose:** The goal of being One, finding the Oneness of everything? How beautiful! And you, Orah, what does living your passion mean to you?

**Orah:** It means keeping a focus on being present and on the Divine, as much as the brain will allow this! This has really been the focus since I got into Ascension. Prior to that, there wasn't much interest in spirituality. I was pretty much a regular guy doing a job as a physiotherapist, father, husband, and member of the community. The spirituality aspect arose pretty much as an epiphany, really. My ex-wife told me she was having a relationship with somebody else and I completely lost the plot. For the first time in my life, I allowed myself to be really angry, allowed myself to scream, and as that was happening, I was watching all these controlling, restrictive, passive aggressive behaviours flash before my eyes. I was watching the way I had controlled things, either in a negative manner, or by being really passive. And through this, there was a realization of a different way of doing Life. I had to find *me.*

It's really difficult, when you're in a relationship that's in crisis, to hang onto a new realization, so I went into a victim role and manically started doing self help courses, just about anything that was going. Then one day, I was in Blackmore's bookshop in Nelson and the proverbial book fell out in front of me, opened at a page, and there was the quote: "The Kingdom of God is within." I realized I needed to stop doing all these courses and trying to find a quick fix, so I stopped everything and began meditating with the same manic intensity! I joined a Zen meditation group and a Taoist meditation group. I also meditated on my own a lot. When I heard about Ascension, it became very clear, within three or four weeks of having done the first Ascension course, I needed to go to North Carolina. I knew there was no choice.

Since then, spirituality has been a nonstop focus. Initially it was very selfish. I just wanted realization for myself! That's really softened quite a lot and I'm much more concerned about other people now. I've realized it's not an individual journey; it has to be a collective thing. The desire has changed to one of wanting everybody to experience unity, and for people to become more aware, so it becomes a process for everybody. Now I integrate that with my work, spending as much time as I can, not necessarily talking about spirituality, but talking about awareness, showing people where they're holding tension in the body, where they're stiff, or where their posture needs improvement. Initially people take an intellectual interest, which eventually can grow to being something more than just coming to the physio for a sore neck, or a sore back, or whatever it happens to be. It seems when people have body complaints or emotional complaints, when they're feeling squeezed, they are more likely to seek assistance and look for more meaning in their lives.

**Rose:** It's bringing the practice of awareness into everyday life, into every meeting. It's just part of who you are?

**Orah:** Yes. The intensity on the self was quite enormous for a number of years, so my passion's changed from being self-focused to being more communal.

**Rose:** I know you met each other through Ascension and the Society for Ascension (SFA) in North Carolina. Can you tell me about that experience?

**Anahata**: It was pretty amazing for me. I continually thank MSI for everything given and graced to me there. It really laid a beautiful foundation as a place to let go and surrender, and for that to become a catalyst for my transformation. I had a spiritual bookstore in Toronto, and this complimentary copy of the book "Ascension" arrived. I was on my way to the Grand Canyon for a Vision Quest. As I stopped by the store on the way to the airport my hand went to this book, and that was it! The book was the only thing I brought with me! By the time I emerged from the Canyon, I knew I was going to North Carolina. No choice! I was being puppeted, driven, led, and divinely guided! When I arrived home, I made a phone call to SFA and when they answered, I burst into tears and said, "I've got to go home! You're my home! That's where I have to be!" Of course my mind was going, "Oh, my God, I'm a single parent, two kids, a business, friends, living at home with my parents." But my heart said, "That's where I have to go!" I made arrangements to do a First Sphere in Asheville and my son came with me. We drove there in one day and arrived two minutes before the start. Before the course was over, I said, "Take me to MSI!" and that was it! We arrived the Sunday night after the weekend was over, I saw MSI, and I knew he would be my future for the next while.

I'd had a very powerful experience five years previously, when I first began work in my store. At the time I was very sick with the flu. It couldn't have gotten any worse and when the children were fighting I yelled at them, "You guys look after yourselves; I'm going into the bedroom." I went and sat on the bed, leaned my back up against the wall and closed my eyes. As I did this, the form of a man appeared, all dressed in black with a white streak through his hair. My heart began beating so intensely, it burst open. The power of it was so strong it flung me back and pinned me to the wall. That's how strong it was. I could barely breathe. As I looked at this man he said, "Everything is going to be all right." As he said that, he put his hand on my left shoulder. As I felt the physical pressure of the hand on my shoulder, I opened my eyes, and thought, "Oh my God, he's here!" Of course, when I opened my eyes, the room was empty. I quickly closed my eyes so I could see him again, but he was gone. The energy of this experience stayed with me over those five years, but it wasn't until I was driving towards Asheville, towards the first First Sphere of Ascension, it dropped into my consciousness:, "Oh my God, that vision was MSI!" As soon as I saw him I knew. It was a sign way back then, I guess, of being prepared energetically to take in that intensity of love. I really needed to be stroked on my body and my consciousness and my willingness to accept that level of love. I was quite a scared bunny prior to this; controlling and controlled, very serious and reserved, really needing to be shaken up!

**Rose:** It sounds like a VERY powerful experience. Was it scary or was there no room for fear?

**Anahata:** It was very, very powerful. Probably one of the most powerful experiences I've had, and no, not scary. I just knew it was true: there *are* very beautiful ascended beings. I knew that's what I had seen. I had been reading spiritual books for some time and this experience set it all in place and made me go into a state of allowing: "Ok, I know this can be true now" and I just opened up to that. That was the fall of 1996.

**Rose:** You were intuitively connected many years before you met MSI in the physical?

**Anahata:** When I bought my New Age bookstore five years previously, I knew nothing about spirituality. I'd never meditated. I bought into this store with eleven others and learned gradually through my customers. I found myself saying things like, "Just witness your thoughts." Watching my thoughts was a very powerful source for knowing myself. But that wasn't me; that wisdom was coming through me. It was a stronger energy. Even though I didn't know where it was leading, or what it was about, it felt very comfortable, natural, real, and like home.

**Rose:** Your connection with MSI was a homecoming! Tell me more about your experience of being with MSI, and at the Centre.

**Anahata:** I'll briefly talk about it, because Orah never met him. Our teacher training was from the fall of '96 to August '97. We, and the group before us, were the only ones who experienced MSI, because he passed in August '97. That was truly, truly amazing and a privilege. I got to experience being in the presence of someone who was unconditionally loving. Yet that unconditional love didn't always show itself as being cuddly. It was Truth! Pure, unconditional truth and love exhibited all the time, for each individual's needs. For instance, some individuals may have appeared to be treated harshly, yet you could still feel the love coming through with the harshness. For others who really needed softness, that aspect came out. If you were willing to see him as Truth, you got to see him as unconditional love all the time.

**Rose**: Was part of that unconditional love a ruthless compassion?

**Anahata**: Yes and his whole life was totally 100% for us. Watching him deal with a cancer in his throat was pretty amazing too, as was watching the reactions and responses of the people around him. For the people who were healers, it brought out a wanting to fix him. I didn't have healing energy in me then and I saw him as a pure being having an experience of cancer, but I knew that wasn't him. For some reason, I saw him as an enlightened man, rather than a sick human. Even on his death bed, when he had no fluids left in his body, he was still exuding amazing, powerful, enlightened energy continuously.

**Rose:** Did he have a specific vision for humanity?

**Anahata:** Yes, he actually saw the energy of enlightenment spreading all around the world. He talked about the 64,000 being the critical point. 64,000 enlightened individuals could transform the whole planet! He always encouraged us to act with integrity. When we went into the homes of people who were sponsoring a course, he said, "You dress well, you behave well, and you leave their home in better condition than when you arrived." He wanted us to be always in service, no matter what went down! He wanted to make sure we were prepared for whatever conditions and behavior were exhibited in our presence, and that we could handle it by sending back love or mirroring back compassion, so they could help themselves.

**Rose:** Both of you became teachers of Ascension?

**Anahata:** Yes.

**Orah:** My path wasn't as clear cut as Anahata's. When I went to North Carolina, I was primarily interested in having time out, so I could better understand myself. When I got there, they talked about this "enlightenment stuff" and it really didn't resonate strongly with me. My brain didn't quite comprehend it. I'd been part of a men's group and some pretty strong hurly burly went on at times; you had to be honest about your emotions. At SFA, most of the meetings were much like that. It was one ongoing group process. There were forty of us, men and women, learning to be with all the various emotions that came up in the course of healing and living together. That was probably the initial highlight for me. I wasn't committed to being a teacher; I was there really just to explore myself. I still had lots of financial limitations and I couldn't see how I was going to make money to meet the ongoing financial requirements for the kids, and so on. It really wasn't until the last minute of the last day it became clear what needed to happen was for me to become a teacher. It was only when I was talking with one of the teachers I realized I'd moved such a long way in terms of how I viewed the world; I couldn't go back and be a regular physio and a regular member of the community. I'd spent such a lot of time experiencing this stuff, now I needed to help pass it on. That's when I made the shift to recognizing I was part of a collective process. I changed.

**Rose:** How long were you at SFA?

**Orah:** Ten months, and for seven of those months I had my eyes closed. I was a slow poke! I used to think a lot and you can't get there by thinking! It took me a long time to allow the flow of things to come through and to realize thinking really was something that happened to me, it wasn't the essence of me, or something that could be relied upon as a method of living. I realized the brain or "thinkingness" is not really who I am, and that was the piece I needed to pass on to others. I come from a background of being reasonably intellectual and rational, so my path has been one of trusting. I've had to learn to trust that what I experience and what I know are the key pieces. The essence is not the ongoing commentary to my life, or any of the thoughts and feelings which happen to pass through.

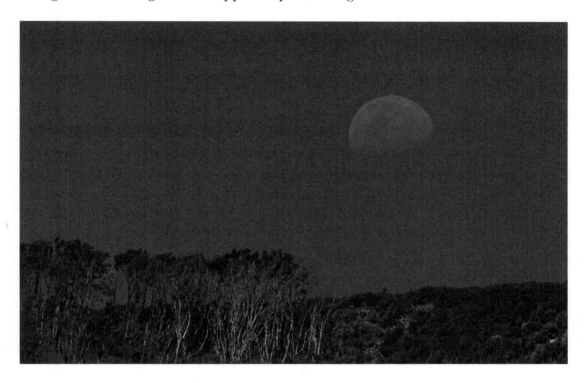

**Rose:** You said, "You can't get there by thinking." Where is it you want to get to?

**Orah:** The place of finding one's essence or Higher Self, or whatever you want to call it. You can't experience that unless you become a little bit separated from the thinking mind. It isn't until you can begin to see the endless flow of the conceptual mind, you realize there's a hell of a lot more than "thinkingness" and logic and all the "stuff" schools, universities, and most of society are focused on. By experiencing gaps in that "thinkingness" I realized it actually flowed past me or through me, or I experienced it as an ongoing changing pattern, rather than being totally engrossed in the thinking and the emotions.

**Rose:** As the thinking cleared away, you connected more with essence?

**Orah**: Yes, I started to experience an awareness of my essence while all this other "stuff" was going on. That awareness comes and goes. I lose it and then it comes back more clearly. I still do ongoing study for the physio registration and, when I was writing various essays, I realized there's a distinction between recognizing and knowing. There's much more than the manifestation of the physical; whether it is moving or running or feeling or talking or being intimate, whatever it happens to be. There's an underlying essence there, and that is what life is all about.

**Rose:** The goal is to be in essence all the time, whatever's going on around you?

**Orah**: Yes, it's an experience and I think there are many people who don't experience it as clearly as they are able to intellectualize it.

**Rose:** When you left SFA and came back out into the world as teachers, after very powerful and deep experiences of both meditation and intense emotional clearing within a group, was it a big adjustment to come back into the world?

**Orah**: For me, it was more difficult, because I got hooked into the idea that a spiritual experience could only be obtained in isolation, when removed from society, and/or sitting with legs crossed, with the hands in the right mudra! I still hadn't moved on to spirituality being something that's active and happening and dynamic every minute of the day. With Ascension, you have attitudes you use all the time, which are intended for use in the world, but in my mind, I still held the idea of the monk sitting in a holy, spiritual place. This concept softened and changed, to realizing spirituality is happening all the time and all I have to do is be content with it as it flows. It really has been a quest to bring that practice forward so everybody can experience it all the time. You don't have to find a special bit of bush, or a special place in the house. You don't have to remove yourself from life in order to manage your life better. You don't have to sit down and meditate for half an hour, three times a day. You can cope with life every second as it comes. Ultimately, the goal is less esoteric: it is to experience causeless joy and love, and this happens when the thinking mind is de-clutched from experiencing the senses.

**Rose**: Connecting with essence *is* a discipline. It *is* a practice. It *is* a constant remembrance. It can happen within the context of an ordinary everyday life!

## Becoming non-duality in every moment

**Anahata:** It became very clear with Ascension, if you were a teacher; you wanted to return to SFA. We lived there and went out from there every weekend to teach all over the USA. We moved to Mexico after Orah graduated; I had been teaching for about four years at that point. We set up house with some other teachers in Mexico, and I was there for thirteen months and Orah, maybe eight or nine months. We went all over Mexico teaching and, as we got to see the same people a lot, we became part of their world and reality. It was different from going for a weekend, meeting people, and then never seeing them again. It put things in a different perspective; we became part of each of those communities and part of the community we were living in. All of a sudden, it became clear to me it wasn't about going back to SFA anymore. By then, it had split in two anyway. We had to start becoming non-duality in every moment. So one step after another, we ended up coming here to Nelson. Ascension didn't take off here in a big way and I realized we didn't even necessarily have to be teaching meditation, we simply had to have the flow of our life as the vehicle for our meditation. We really slowed down on our own personal meditation. Instead, we started to see our experiences, and our meetings with people and the events that happened in our lives, as a whole moving meditation.

*James: A Caring seed*

*If I could sow a seed for a new world, I would sow a Caring seed. The whole world would be Caring for each other with no fighting or drugs. The whole world would be clean and if someone hurt themself someone would always come and help. Countries wouldn't need the Police or the Army. Everybody would be friends, people could play games with each other e.g. a Boy playing with a Girl without their friends laughing at them or calling them names. People wouldn't get carried away playing games then hurting someone else.*

**Rose:** Do you think there was a purpose to you being called to Nelson?

**Anahata**: We were in Sydney and were going to set up shop there, with Orah working as a physio. We had just gotten married and, because

I only had a three month visa, I had to leave the country. I ended up teaching for a month in New Zealand and Samyamah found out I was in the country and asked me to come to Nelson. She picked me up at the airport and, as we drove around Rocks Road, I said,"Oh my God, this is my place!"

I had seen this place in my mind for years and years, even in my teens, so it was very noticeable when we got here; this is where we needed to be. People started asking us to stay, and then we had a four day advanced training with a group of twenty people, which was like an anchoring. I was in the middle of an expansion, a unity experience at the time. When I went back to Sydney, Orah picked me up at the airport, and I said, "Honey, I have something to tell you! I think we need to move to the sweet little town of Nelson!" And he said,"Oh, my God!" That was the Nelson of his life, where he'd left lots of history and had an ex-wife and children. But he knew in his heart, he had to come back here.

**Orah**: That was September 11th; the towers were falling in the U.S. when she delivered this news! It was a time of change, not just in New York!

**Anahata:** That was that! And here's the funny thing: Orah had just made arrangements for all the physio equipment he'd had in storage for three years, to be shipped over on a boat, and when I arrived at the airport, the boat was just pulling into port in Sydney! When we arrived home, there was a letter in the mail from the landlord, which said, "I've sold the house. You have to get out in two weeks!" So within two weeks, I had everything of the little bit we owned, packed up, and I was over here in Nelson.

**Rose:** What is the attraction of Nelson?

**Anahata:** I don't think its Nelson itself, it's just "this is the place!" This is where the energy was pointing to, and it just happens to be a beautiful place with amazing people and energy.

**Rose:** I think Nelson is a spiritual place, as is the whole of the top of the South Island, Nelson and Golden Bay.

**Anahata:** Yes and spiritual Masters have been here too to share. It's definitely a meeting point of spiritual energies.

**Rose:** Tell me a bit about how you got involved with Deeksha and what that has meant to you.

**Orah:** Anahata saw a photo of Sandra and Daniel Biskind, who are Deeksha givers here in New Zealand, and she said: "This woman's got something!" So we went along and received our first Deeksha with them. I didn't experience very much that first time. It was just a nice meditation. I didn't think a lot more of it, but then Daniel said: "Why don't you come to India and experience it?" Because I hadn't settled here very well, I was quite happy to go away yet again. But financially it was a non-starter, as we'd just started the business, so we didn't think about it much more. However, Samyamah went to India and that lit the desire in us again. I came home early one day and was not very happy about the focus of my life and where it was going. I sat down and did some meditation. I'm not prone to visions, but in this meditation I experienced MSI, and he said: "You've been doing really well, but you need to go to India." Within weeks of this meditation, I received a message from relatives in Holland saying one of my aunts, whom I'd never really met, had died and left a certain amount of money. When the money came through it was exactly enough for both of us to go to India, do the course, and pay for a month's rent! The rest is pretty much history.

## Surrendering to joy

The passing on of the desire for expanded consciousness can happen now more effectively through the hands, rather than from just sitting. I get told endlessly that people who aren't meditators suddenly start witnessing; something that took months to establish with Ascension. We've heard people describe incredible unity experiences and huge epiphanies, right down to really simple stories like getting financial "stuff" sorted without even trying. The power of Deeksha is huge! It makes the expansion of consciousness so much more accessible, especially if people are prepared enough, and trusting enough, to let us put our hands on their heads. This implies surrender. With meditation, there's still a control: "I'm doing this." With Deeksha, you surrender, and you then receive what it is you're ready to surrender to. It's really quite a beautiful process.

**Anahata:** Deeksha turns the process of life into an ongoing movie of realizations. You get to witness each thought, feeling, sensation and outward observation, upclose and personal. It takes out the dullness and perks you up into really acknowledging what is truly being presented to you on your buffet table of experiences. The more allowing you are, the more you see. All of life is simply about "seeing", until one day you are de-clutched from the hold of the mind, and dawn into the silent, still consciousness, experiencing the movement. Emotions and thoughts still arise, but they pass like a bird in flight and disappear effortlessly. Joy starts to build and evolves into your normal state of balance, with bliss coming and going. Gratitude grows exponentially to be the only outward energy you want to express, and Life goes on!!!

**Rose:** This certainly sounds very wonderful and something to aspire to! It seems Deeksha is an accelerated process; it changes consciousness more quickly than Ascension did. That seems to me to be connected with the time we're in: things are speeding up.

**Anahata:** Absolutely! Ascension was good for us at that time. It was TM for the time before. The whole focus from the Divine has been in stages, and is evolving as well. Now the mass consciousness is ready for something like the Oneness Blessing.

**Rose:** I believe Bhagavan's and Amma's vision is for enough people to become enlightened to shift mass consciousness?

**Orah:** It's the 64,000 again.

**Anahata:** They've said one person who is enlightened affects over 100,000 people, anywhere in the world. I'm starting to understand the energy that flows through each one of us and how we're interlinked and I can see how that happens very easily.

**Rose:** How do you see this evolving? Are you confident and optimistic the collective shift is going to happen?

**Anahata:** I don't know that anybody, even Bhagavan, can say it's going to happen. But there are events happening all over the world, like "Fire the Grid." Even 9/11 started to bring forth compassion; the tsunami too. You can't hold any one thing in isolation. We truly are One Heart, and our One-Heartedness is manifesting in all sorts of events, varieties of therapy, movements, and beautiful spiritual awakenings. We can only keep holding the vision it's going to keep getting better. In any process of healing, there is always some mucky "stuff", isn't there? When a glass is full of junk at the bottom, the junk has to rise and it's murky for a while. If you keep the water flowing, it clears. That's what's happening for consciousness. We just have to allow the murky bits to come forth, because they've been solid and holding fast for such a long time. We should be celebrating the fact they're there, and floating, and coming forward; it means the energy is being freed.

**Rose:** It's like flushing out the toxins from the social body.

**Anahata:** It's coming from the micro to the macro. We have to allow the flow of it all.

## A place of nonsuffering

**Orah:** A final comment to:"are things happening?" I guess the answer is yes! We've had four people in Nelson who have moved on to a place of nonsuffering. We know there are more in Byron Bay and we've heard there are more still in Europe and the States. That's pretty much unprecedented in history! As far as we know, there have never been these numbers of people in this higher state. That's what keeps me saying: "Yes, things are moving in the right direction. " It gives me hope. Amma and Bhagavan say, they set the stage for enlightenment, joy and bliss to happen, but they're not the ones who make the final call. It is a Source beyond them that pulls the strings. The process is happening whether you follow Ammabhagavan, or Buddhism, or Christianity, or any other path.

**Anahata:** I want to thank you very much Rose, for doing your part in the collective transformation. As we share our hearts like this, we are actually igniting our evolution even more! The visualisations, heart's desires, the selfless service, as we share all of this, it raises the global resonance like a catalyst. The suffering of mankind will be an event in a past sphere of existence. The Golden Age of Peace will bring us so much more to experience. But first we all have to become free and know we are One.

# Creating
# New Models

## *We are part of a global movement*

There are millions of people all over the world working to create new ways of being and living together which honour the multidimensional nature of human life. Many have been working patiently, and often with very little reward, for years, even decades. In the past, we have been called "counter-cultural", living in reaction to the mainstream values of society. Now, instead of being in angry reaction to the old ways, we are simply withdrawing our energy and attention from ways which are not working, to focus instead, with love and commitment, on the conscious choice to live in joyful service to creating new ways, alongside the old. This shift from removing attention from what is not working, to putting our full attention on what we choose and intend to create, is pivotal in the process of transformation and profoundly liberating for all who make it.

When we withdraw our attention and energy from what is not working and choose to focus on allowing our creative being to unfold and flow into form, we stop seeing people and social structures as needing to be fixed, and instead simply go ahead to develop new models of being together in relationship, community, and business. In this way, a new world based on the new evolutionary consciousness begins to emerge alongside the old one. The people and projects in this book offer some possible ways forward and will hopefully stimulate some questions and answers in you.

Right now, I am sitting amidst my own questions. I am in the United States as I write this, and there are rumours of the fall of the US economy and impending global economic collapse. Yesterday, I heard two major finance companies have crashed in New Zealand. A few years ago, while visiting family in England, there was a strike by the truck drivers who deliver petrol to gas stations. It quickly became apparent how fragile the infrastructure of our Western urban consumer society is, and how easily the everyday life we take for granted could be disrupted. How will millions of people living in urban conurbations survive when the oil runs out? What damage is being sustained by the Earth as a consequence of depleting oil stocks? How is it, with all our scientific and technological inventiveness, there aren't many alternative fuels already available? What will happen if food can no longer be delivered to supermarkets? What if we can no longer drive our cars to shop? Although peak oil is now in the collective consciousness, how often do we really stop and think about it, let alone make any preparations for living in a different way? Last night we had one of many violent thunderstorms and lost our supply of electricity for several hours. We are having a taste of what's in store with global warming as we suffer a hot, humid summer in which electric fans and air conditioning are essential for well-being. How will we manage if the power goes out and doesn't come on again? How can we prepare and take action rather than waiting for crises to hit? What does it take for humanity to wake up and start doing things differently? I am one of a growing multitude of voices asking these questions.

As I'm writing, news drops into my inbox of two movies which corroborate the fragility of our ecosystem. "A CRUDE AWAKENING" is a documentary feature film about how we are sucking our non-renewable oil reserves dry and how dangerously close we are to the bottom of the barrel. "THE ELEVENTH HOUR" is based on interviews with leading experts in the fields of ecology, public policy, social critique and visionary philosophy. It provides an overview of the technology, politics and consequences of corporate and consumer behaviour, and the aspirations and means to fix the mess we've created.

The "eleventh hour" refers to the last moment when change is possible before it's too late to do anything. The message of both these films is that we've reached a limit point in our collective affairs, when we are imposing such strain on our ecosystem, it could collapse, together with our economic and power systems. Denial may have served us well in keeping fear and panic at bay, but it has also kept us blind, powerless and unresponsive. Ongoing denial and self interest continue unabated. On my walk this morning, I noticed numerous driveways

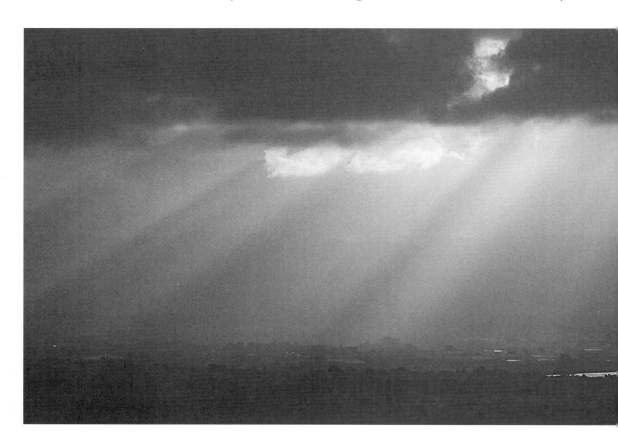

with two or three vehicles parked in them and many gas-guzzling SUV's. Nor do I feel personally exempt from self interest. I'd love to be free to keep travelling on airplanes between the US and New Zealand, so I can be in the land I love and maintain my relationship with Woods in America. Although I'm well aware of the environmental impact of jumbo jet travel, it is difficult to voluntarily surrender such privileges, even when I know how toxic they are. Last night I read an interesting observation which caused me to further reflect on how much we take for granted in our comfortable Western life styles: "If everyone in China and India used toilet paper, every tree in the world would be gone in a year." (1)

We walk a thin line between denial on the one hand and fear on the other. How can we stay awake and aware of the realities, yet at the same time, avoid falling into fear-based reactions which push us back into duality, separation and scarcity thinking? The people in this book put their focus on choosing to maintain consciousness in the highest

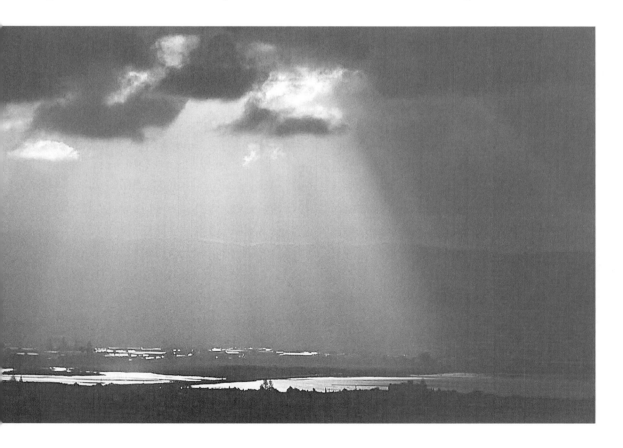

possible state; making their best contribution through living their passion; taking actions to make their lives more eco-friendly; starting to envision and build the new emerging culture by developing ways of living co-creatively. Beyond that, research suggests that intentional group meditation may correlate with reduced violence and crime in a given area. (2) Participating in weekly global meditations for peace would, I believe, strengthen the field of peaceful consciousness around the planet.

## Community is our most valuable resource

What would a more eco-friendly and communal society look like? My experience in New Zealand is helpful with this. The top of the South Island is inhabited by many people who, like me, are looking for a relaxed, unpretentious lifestyle with easy access to wild nature. Although there are plenty of wealthy people in the area, on the whole there isn't a great deal of cash flowing. Along with many others, I learned to simplify my life and live without the frills and luxuries I'd taken for granted in Scotland. This didn't seem a great sacrifice as my quality of life was very good. Many people I know build their own attractive, quirky and original houses, using low impact materials, such as mud bricks and straw bales, installing solar panels and composting toilets. They plant gardens and orchards. They keep washing machines, cars, and other appliances for decades rather than trading them in for the latest model. They wear recycled clothes and look fabulous. When I lived in Edinburgh we would go to a rock concert, the opera, or the theatre for entertainment, whereas in Nelson and Golden Bay we make our own entertainment within a vibrant participatory community. Whereas in the past, people flocked to church for their sense of belonging, now we find it in heart-sharing circles and gatherings, where we explore subjective experience, dance barefoot on the earth and play drums beneath the stars.

Such experiences, amongst many others, have taught me to value community. The publicity for "A Crude Awakening" speaks of oil as being our most valued and non-renewable resource. Certainly, it appears to some to be a resource worth killing for. What if the exhaustion of the world's oil supplies is a gift we have given ourselves to motivate us to discover new values and solutions? What if the end of petrol driven vehicles, whilst highly "inconvenient" for humanity, turns out to be a blessing in disguise? I remember a time back in the nineties when, at the beginning of my soul journey, I wrote-off my car through a minor accident. I was living in the far North West Highlands of Scotland, where there was no public transport and very little traffic. Until that point, I would have deemed it inconceivable I could survive there without my own individual "bubble of independence". However, I learned to take buses, cycle and hitchhike, and this brought me more in touch with people and nature. If there was no bus and nobody stopped to pick me up, I simply didn't go wherever I felt I "had to" go; I trusted the synchronicity and survived just fine. I began to realize how my car had contributed to an illusion of independence and freedom, which cut me off from others, just as the good income I'd previously commanded as a psychotherapist, gave me the illusion I could have whatever I wanted and go wherever I wanted, without needing others. My affluence robbed me of the experience of interconnectedness and interdependence; foundation-stones of community. Needless to say, this was frequently a lonely and empty existence, from which I was delivered by my longing for more human and spiritual sustenance. In my first year in New Zealand, I spent four months walking around the South Island on a peace walk. Since we had very little money, I learned how to ask for support and to understand the mutual flow of give and take that creates relationship and community. Once again, I discovered how much more alive and connected I felt when I was actually in contact with nature, rather than rushing through it in my bubble of steel. I meet many people in Western society who are trapped in similarly compulsive independence, believing if they have enough money, enough property, enough goods, they will somehow be "secure" and fulfilled. In our culture, we have become dependent on cars and built our lives around them. Personally, I find the idea of a "car free" world has many advantages: clean air, freedom from noise pollution and the healing of the planet, being uppermost. If we weren't so busy rushing around, we might discover an inner stillness, and be surprised by the realization that everything we need is right here where we are.

I am envisioning a world where people wake up to the urgency of our situation and voluntarily agree to give up driving cars for two years. It wouldn't take so long to organize an efficient public transport system and reorganize shopping. Within two years, human inventiveness would discover any number of eco-friendly alternatives to oil. I'm sure this will sound far-fetched, idealistic and inconceivable to some readers, and it certainly would have to be a collective choice, but think about it! What is it going to take for us to stop the insanity of our present destructive way of life? Will it take a catastrophe for us to join together?

A couple of days after writing this, I heard China has declared its first"car free" day, closely followed by San Francisco! How wonderful it would be to have days without cars, lawn mowers or power tools! Days of peace, and how simple!

I contend, rather than oil being our most valued resource, our most valuable resource is community, and community is a renewable resource. Moving from an experience of individual isolation, to a realization of interconnectedness and interdependence, is vitally important to our collective well-being and survival. Developing community is central; whether this is in specific localities; in business; between policy makers, academics, scientists and grassroots projects; across cultures, races, and religions; or in bringing experiential learning communities together around specific themes.

What sorts of communities will we grow as we step into the future? How might we bring our human resource of scientific and technological brilliance into harmony with nature, and in service to a vision of One World?

The people in this next section provide examples of community initiatives, which I hope will open up a sense of some of the possibilities in you.

**Daring Donna:** Many labels have been given to what Daring Donna and a group of extraordinary, innovative beings have been holding and doing: Co-creative Work Community; Co-creators; Open Space Community. However, DD likes to see it simply as "Love-in-action", without rules, guidelines, structure, or even a long term vision. She talks here about the practice of co-creation and how she is facilitating this process in local communities, and in business. One such community event, "The Great New Zealand Street Party", will bring people together locally throughout New Zealand on February 23 '08. The simple intention behind this is to bring people out of their houses and onto the streets to say hello, chat with each other and celebrate being alive; a fun way to plant seeds and open the way for community to flourish. Donna talks also about business initiatives built around the process of co-creation, which go beyond the idea of "yours and mine" to share resources, skills and profits. This book is one such project.

**Robin Allison** is an architect who took the inspiring initiative to create Earthsong Eco-Neighbourhood in the suburbs of Auckland. Based on ideas from the co-housing movement, Earthsong is a New Zealand first, which has brought together a group of householders on a few acres. When I visited Earthsong in 2000, it was an apple orchard. Revisiting in 2007, the orchard had been transformed into a beautiful haven, hidden away behind the busy road, with spacious rammed earth houses, gardens abundant with flowers and vegetables, and a gracious common house. One of the greatest losses of late 20th and early 21st century life has to be the loss of meaning and belonging that accompanies the breakdown of neighbourhood. Earthsong is a fine example of what can be achieved through co-operative housing, which in this case, is also low impact and eco-friendly. Robin has held and focused the vision for thirteen years, working with a group to bring it into being. A wariness of leadership appears to be an inherent part of the independent, pioneering, "Kiwi" psyche and I was particularly interested in exploring how Robin had managed hers.

**Margaret Jefferies:** Sustainability is at the heart of many initiatives for grassroots change. Margaret Jefferies and Wendy Everingham have been working for the last three years with the goal of turning their community of 3000 people in Lyttelton, near Christchurch, into a more vibrant, sustainable town. This is a voluntary initiative which started small and has built considerable momentum, touching the lives of many individuals and groups within the community, and beyond.

Project Port Lyttelton now includes a thriving farmers market, a time share system for exchanging skills without money, a waste minimisation scheme, a local newspaper, and community festivals; all of which serve to bring people together into co-creative relationships, which support the wealth and well-being of the whole community. This project has been fostered mostly by just two special, committed people, who had the courage to live their passion and seize opportunities. The success of Project Port Lyttelton is now opening the way for bigger conversations, bringing diverse interest groups together into alliances that will affect future directions for the whole community, and influence decision makers at local government and ministerial levels. This is a wonderful example of grassroots, bottom-up social transformation and they have won a civic award for their work.

**James Samuel** shares a similar vision for Waiheke Island, near Auckland. He talks about the importance of empowering communities to make decisions, share resources and meet needs locally. Spaces in which people can come together for dialogue and trust-building, can act as containers and attractor fields for building co-creative community. The whole can then be further supported through developing a vibrant community hub and using computer technology to link people with services such as a car sharing.

**Robina McCurdy** is a founding member of the Tui Community, an intentional community in Golden Bay which has been developing its own strong earth-based culture for over twenty years. Robina is an expert in developing sustainable community and living in harmony with the land through permaculture. She is also a gifted facilitator of community, guiding groups to bring their visions into reality. Here, she describes how she and her partner, Huckleberry, brought together a learning community around the building of their mud brick home, according to the principles of deep sustainability. Our conversation turned to a discussion of how a co-creative community can tune into the flow of life and manifest from that flow, imbuing their task with a sense of the sacred. I first met Robina when I was staying at Tui community twelve years ago; she had just returned from a work trip in South Africa, to be greeted by a pod of dolphins swimming in the bay!

Since then I have watched, and at times participated in, the evolution of her work, as she untiringly lives her passion as a transformational catalyst and guardian of Gaia.

**Daniel Batten:** Having already become a successful entrepreneur, Daniel is now able to divide his time between business and his life purpose, teaching "The Art of Living", a spiritual practice which uses the breath to control the fear based aspect of mind, so that life may be experienced more fully. Here, he describes a business model based on nature's abundance and the rhythm of the breath, which encourages entrepreneurs to give back to communities, as they create wealth. Acting as a bridge between the business world and a spiritual way of living, Daniel combines business acumen and pragmatism with higher, spiritual values such as love, generosity and interdependence. Most people who choose to live their passion experience fear from time to time. I have met Daniel in several different roles and contexts. My favourite experience was in a theatre improvisation group he ran at Swanson Sanctuary. Not only did he create an environment in which I could step through a lifelong fear of anything theatrical, but I watched with delight Daniel's graceful and playful flow of improvisation, seeing the creative process in action, flowing through him, unimpeded by self consciousness or fear.

**Leanne Holdsworth:** Rather than belonging to any one community, Leanne is like a bee cross-pollinating gardens, as she follows her passionate mission for social justice and social responsibility through the corporate world and with policy makers. After focusing her energy and influence to help make corporate environments more humane, Leanne understood the need for a simple process to enable people to explore what community means to them, and to take steps to build it in their workplaces and neighbourhoods. In response to this need, she created The Caring Communities Project. Leanne is now extending her work to bring multi-disciplinary decision makers together in deeper conversations, encouraging them to connect more closely with the real everyday needs of the people they are serving. Once again I was struck by how much one visionary and focused individual can achieve.

These are just a few examples of innovative thinking and action; a handful of evolutionary seeds. They are creative experiments in whole system community living. I hope they will inspire individuals, policy makers and philanthropists to see a more creative way forward into the future.

# TRANSFORMING COMMUNITY

## Living our passion as Love-in-action is a way of service

The beauty of it is, living our passion serves the good of the larger whole. When we choose to live our passion, we do what is essentially ours to do: our soul work. When we do what we love to do wholeheartedly, from a place of authenticity and integrity, combining our passion with skill and commitment, in alignment with our highest values and for the good of all, we support the evolution of humanity, and we are in turn supported.

These interviews clearly show, when we do work we really love, work that stretches us into creative freedom and connects us in meaningful relationship and community, such a sense of fulfillment arises, we need very little more to satisfy us. The lust for material goods and power which drives the world's troubles is, at least in part, a compulsion to fill the emptiness we experience when the realization of our essential nature and the interconnectedness of life is lost, or not yet developed. Many people in this book aim to live simplified lives, yet paradoxically, when they express the emerging new spirit of personal and social transformation, and live in service to it, their lives become more meaningful and filled with true abundance, magic, and flow.

# Living your Passion means:

*We simply do what excites us, what makes our hearts sing, what we have fun doing. We have understood what is, imagined what could be, and are co-creating what will be, to "be the change" we feel in our hearts. —Donna*

*This one life I have is possibly all I will ever have, and the world really needs us to be as aware, as connected, and as intentional as possible. For me, that means nothing actually matters except making sure this planet's going to survive. —Robin*

*The creative spirit is relentless and it keeps on going! As soon as something's created, you don't sit back, relax, and say wow, the next thing comes on! I'm allowing myself to do what touches my heart, to be bold and ask questions. —Margaret*

*If there's one thing that focuses my energy, it's this thing of localization: meeting our needs and making decisions locally through self government, local food production, information sharing, dialogue, creative housing/shelter solutions, and creative uses of land. —James*

*Living my passion means not compromising what motivates me forward into action. My passion is social change, environmental restoration and contributing energy to turn around a situation for the betterment of the whole. —Robina*

*What does it mean to live in a way which is empowered, empowering and acknowledging of some of the problems that are in the world at the moment, in a way that doesn't go into either denial or despair, but gives us a container of hope and joy, exhilaration and challenge? —Daniel*

*For me it's about influencing; the underlying thing that always drives my passion is fairness and my response to injustice. —Leanne*

# *Shift Nine*

## From separation, to building sustainable, co-creative community wherever we happen to be.

Recognizing the power of grassroots change, and the necessity for us all to learn to live together and get along, we begin to create community wherever we are. Opportunities arise for accelerated creativity and learning, mutual support, conscious relationship, and sharing resources. We accept the challenge to bring forth new attitudes, skills, and creative solutions to humanity's problems.

# Daring Donna
## Welcome everyone to the Garden!

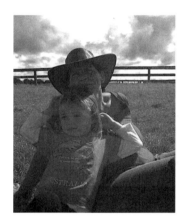

Since I was a very wee girl, I have been guided to "be the change I wanted to see in the world" and this has taken various forms. Living on the land with a tight knit family of four gave me a deep understanding of nature's cycles and what it means to live in community. I love Aotearoa and feel very at home on the lands of this beautiful country. Being able to explore my own creativity freely from a young age, has led to some wonderful opportunities which have included a stint as a sports person paddling kayak for New Zealand, playing women's rugby and winning gold medals in surf lifesaving. I owned a successful adventure company and worked with some big multinational companies, both here and in England. However, my greatest achievements are the conscious, beautiful, loving relationships I have created with my partner of nine years, Darren and my family and friends, who have travelled many roads with me. Thousands of hours of community work and service; beach clean-ups; youth programmes; community visioning, events and festivals; food and shelter for those in need; animal rescue and community gardens; have helped to shape my experience and opened many doors. I now find myself again working outside the "tape worm" system for the betterment of all in Aotearoa. In May 2005, while looking after one of my gorgeous nieces full time for my beloved sister and brother, I was guided to meet a visiting Brazilian visionary, Eduardo Araujo and together with Anne Curtis, spent the rest of the year dialoguing and experimenting with co-creation. This has now become practical in the form of a co-creating work community with people coming together in a variety of co-created projects: Circus Schmirkus, The Great New Zealand Street Party, Open Arted, Rose Coloured Glasses, Caring Communities. The experiment of co-creation has also manifested Swanson Sanctuary, a physical space for meeting, living, working and playing, on an eight acre property under the Waitakere Ranges. www.streetparty.co.nz

**Donna:** I resonate to live in the flow and serve for the good of all. I find when I am living my passion I am calm within and feel much love, joy, peace and harmony everywhere, in everything. For me "living my passion" is about being heart centred and not fear controlled.

Since I was little it's always been about Love-in-action, doing things with great love because I can and they resonate with me. It's never been about me, about self, but whenever self does arise, I know I'm living the illusion of separation, which is part of our collective consciousness at this time in humanity's evolution. Love, laugh, live I say!

Letting go of self, and connecting with infinite consciousness, is the only way for me to lead a fulfilling life, lived in passion. When I'm not listening, I feel it immediately in my solar plexus; I get blocked up. My body, my head and the people around me all let me know.

Living my passion is not even about what I do. What I do is somewhat irrelevant. If I have that connection with Source, I feel joy, happiness, love and freedom; that calm space within me. That's living my passion! I could drive a truck, sweep floors, prune trees, have the biggest publishing company in the world, or grow organic food. It wouldn't matter what I did! Living my passion only happens when I'm connected and serving my highest good, which is ultimately humanity's highest good. Trying to convey this in words is a little beyond the English language. *Laughter.* So in a nutshell: "It's not all about me!"

When I was young I wanted to help save the world, then I wanted to help heal the world and now there's no big vision. I'm very much going with the flow of spirit and being of service. I know in my whole body, heart and soul, that the world is about to change. I've been waiting for the change a long time and I feel very excited. If I went into scarcity consciousness, then the change would be quite scary, so I choose to live in a rose-coloured world. As in James Redfield's, *The Celestine Prophecy*, when people focus on the flowers and see their energy, that's how I see the world. I've always seen it that way; the only time I don't is when I jump out of my heart space. Inside I feel peace, freedom, joy, happiness and extreme love.

If I keep my life simple, then everything's sweet. My emotional and physical bodies feel free of much of the old conditioning (thanks to some awesome learning experiences and a great healer) so I feel I can connect with the new energy, as it flows through, very quickly. At the beginning of this year, we set up this "family of co-creators" which is a learning community, and for me, it's a step in humanity's evolution. We've co-created an on-line dialogue tool and a physical setting just out of Auckland in the country. It's a place from which people can do their "Love-in-action" with projects that are in service to the whole. Conscious co-creation is a way forward together in the years to come.

## *Love-in-action means power-with*

**Rose:** I know co-creation and living as Love-in-action are very important to you and motivate the innovations you are bringing into being. Please tell me more about the work you're doing with the network of co-creators.

**Donna**: At this moment in time the world is changing rapidly and it's important to be in the now, to let go of attachments and go with the flow. In practical terms, that means allowing our creativity to flow without placing limits on when, where and how. We have found by creating conscious relationships, taking full responsibility for ourselves, and co-creating in a way of respect for all living things, in mutual support and resource, we have surpassed what we thought was possible.

The current system is out of order. It definitely feels time to let it be, and it will collapse all on its own. Many people are not aware that at this time, some of us have power over us. It's discreet, and we build systems to protect and defend this "power." "Power-over" is a system based in fear. What systems have power over us? Here are some: banks, insurance companies, governments, business, the education system, justice system, services for child, youth and family, the economical system, the trade system, universities, building consent and resource. Maybe this sounds like a sweeping statement? There are more and more movies available now that support this view. Why did "The Matrix" movies become one of the Top 10 grossing movie trilogies of our time? Maybe because we know it, feel it, live it daily! I challenge everyone to have the courage to take their power back, be the best they are right now, and support the good of all!

**Rose:** How do we become "Love-in-action" in the current fear-based system, in which we have been conditioned to give our power away?

**Donna:** All we simply do is "live our passion" and tune in to what excites us, what makes our hearts sing and what we have fun doing! It's about each individual learning to take full responsibility for self: physically, mentally, emotionally, spiritually, and financially; each individual standing in her own power and in his own truth. We seeded a community garden for common unity in mid 2006, where we could do our "Love-in-action", using this concept of co-creation, and mutually supporting and resourcing the whole for the good of all. We have understood what is, imagined what could be, and are co-creating what will be, to "be the change" we feel in our hearts.

After many conversations, gatherings, wanangas, and the building of conscious relationships; we started a few projects to experiment. One such project is Swanson Sanctuary, at the foot of the Waitakere Ranges on the outskirts of Auckland. Here a group of people have been drawn together to evolve new ways of working and doing business co-creatively, embodying Love-in-action. The group moved into Swanson Sanctuary in September 2006, and created a space for meeting, living, working and playing, around the principle of W.E: Welcome Everyone and financed by trust. Using an online project management tool, Basecamp, we are able to work remotely around the country on a huge range of projects, depending on where people's passions lead them, and keep everyone in touch with what's happening.

**Rose:** Having stayed for several weeks at Swanson Sanctuary, the seedbed for many co-creative projects, I know how dynamic and leading edge the practice of co-creating can be. How has it evolved for you?

**Donna:** Once upon a time, seeds of co-creation were planted on Planet Earth. These seeds sprouted in fertile soil, and many around the world saw the beauty in these plants and began to water and weed. In May 2005, a few of us who felt called, organized an event: "Be the Change You Want to See in the World", and then we sat together every Thursday for about eight months, co-creating a way of being and doing in the world to honour all living systems. In June 2006, we took a seed of co-creation from the world's community garden and tended it right here in Aotearoa. We found in co-creation, we could mutually support and resource, take self responsibility and fully express our creativity in ways we could never have done on our own. Co-creation worked and it felt time to share it.

In August 2006, a Co-Creators wananga was held in Auckland with people coming from all over Aotearoa. We discovered through sharing our unity is in service to humanity, Planet Earth, and all living systems. How we service is our diversity.

Every couple of months, when someone is moved to call a wananga, we meet in a sharing circle to connect, listen, learn and inspire. As well as Swanson Sanctuary, many other co-creative living spaces are popping up throughout Aotearoa, in the form of eco-villages, whanau houses and farms, where people can live for a moment, or a longer time, and learn sustainability within community.

We wanted to experiment with the idea of a "Co-creative Work Community" different from the current system, in which we're encouraged to compete against each other through sole trading, partnerships, companies and 'not-for-profits'. We felt the call to mutually support and resource the whole through sustainable business practices and to help individuals express their creativity. We are all so very different and now twelve months down the track, we find over thirteen projects co-created around the country.

**Rose:** There seems to be a desire to create business in a different way, where everyone benefits, and to develop models of business which serve humanity as a whole, as well as the people immediately involved.

**Donna:** I see it even bigger than that. What I see is business, community projects; it's all a garden where we can express our creativity, with vehicles or tools to help us all lift our consciousness. Most of us want to express ourselves fully and so we try to find a space in this world where we can do this. It may be through our work, children, sport, art, writing, partner, social life, or group. What we are learning through co-creating is how to fully express ourselves, while servicing the whole, creating conscious relationships, and being sustainable. It's experiential learning and we don't have all the answers, but we are sure having fun finding out what works and what doesn't! *Laughter.*

## Planting our seeds in the garden of co-creation

**Rose:** The idea of co-creation being a garden, in which everyone plants their seeds, is a vivid symbol for you?

**Donna:** As I see it, we all have a seed. We bring our seed to the garden, and each is very individual, unique and different. We plant our seed into this garden, which has been created for us in fertile ground. People have done a lot of healing and learning, and now we're looking at how to work and live together and be together for the common good, for Mother Earth, Father Sky and all living things. How do we do this in a garden of such vast diversity? Some of the plants need a lot of watering; others are flowering beyond what they ever thought they could. How do we share the bees around?

For me, it doesn't matter all that much what we do. It's how we go about doing it and the learning that comes from this. This learning community welcomes everyone. Who are we to say someone isn't welcome in the garden, if they have the call from spirit to be here? Maybe I don't like cacti, but that's ok, I can hang out with the marigolds! That's what I've noticed with co-creators: souls connect, personalities clash sometimes. That's ok too, but as soon as I sit down in a circle, even if it's a personality I don't fully connect with, as soon as I can look into their eyes and connect with their soul, it's sweet. *Laughter.*

**Rose:** So you're holding a space in which everybody is welcome and trusting that whoever comes into this space is here because they're called here, there's a reason for them to have shown up? They might be here for their own growth or for the lessons that you learn in relation to them. You seem to be saying: what connects us is that we're all human.

**Donna:** Yes, and we're all learning. One of the things we're learning through co-creating is how to be there for each other, so the garden grows into a beautiful, fruitful one for everyone.

**Rose:** So this is a transformational learning community! There's a willingness to step out of old ways and experiment with new ways. At this pivotal time, surely the world needs places like this! Tell me more, Donna, about how you understand the process of co-creating.

**Donna:** The concept of co-creation is very, very simple and also powerful. I'll use the explanation I arrived at with a dear friend Eduardo Manoel Araujo. It's based on the quantum physics concepts, where we know we are part of the whole and interconnected; and the whole is within us. We are part of the Universe and the entire history of the Universe is inside us, physically speaking. Fractal theory shows how the patterns of nature tend to repeat as we start successively zooming into any part. Co-creation is based on this natural phenomenon that science has captured for us. The idea is simply that each part of the community represents, has the identity, and acts as a whole which has all the parts inside it.

So that's the short concept of co-creation and the short process is, everyone brings a kite of gifts, skills, experiences, needs, wants, resources, knowledge, knowing, time, and finds their passion. Together we support and resource the whole for the good of all, while taking full responsibility for ourselves. It is definitely an experiment at present, as we move from the fear-based model of scarcity we have been educated and brainwashed to live, to one of love. One year into co-creation, it sometimes feels as if we have only just begun to learn to let go and trust the flow.

I really do have the sense if we take the leap and go with our inner guidance rather than outside plans, the world will change before our very eyes. It's happening already! I am seeing even in the corporate sector, they are trying to find the heart, as people evolve and make more intuitive decisions in their lives.

## Finding the heart of business through co-creation

**Rose:** Can you give an example of how this is happening?

**Donna:** For many years in the 80's and 90's, I worked in the corporate world, in Human Resources. The consultants, trainers, facilitators and leaders were setting up "self directed work teams", empowering individuals and using mind strategies, incentives and competitions to "make" highly productive work teams, so that profit to shareholders grew and grew and grew.

Now we see "senior management" teams seeking help to find the heart of the business, becoming more holistic and collaborative in their approach to leadership, and people actually demanding a balance of work and life when they apply for new roles.

We are evolving, and co-creation is another tool in the evolutionary process. Many tools have been used before and many more will come later.

**Rose:** You see co-creating as a new model for the future. How do you see the old business model and the shift to the new?

**Donna**: In my first twenty years of adulthood I always worked to time lines, usually someone else's or I set my own. It's interesting how, in the last four or five years, I seem to have done just as much as I did in the first twenty, but without the time constraints and stress. I also find as I engage with more people, a lot of what I used to do single handed gets done by many and thus feels more enjoyable.

I see it in terms of a distribution flow on the web of life. As we remember the flow of life and let go of old behaviours, beliefs, conditioning, and the desire to control and step into our truth; we enter the flow of life. We are all connected, tiny lights shining on a huge web of life that is interconnected. We can feel its power when we sit together or alone in quiet reflection, meditation, or prayer. We more often than not lose this connection with the web of life when we step into doing. When we understand this natural connection and flow, we can really look and feel into how we connect into this web and how we lose our connection.

If something comes through from Source into the imagination as an idea, it's definitely then time to feel into it and go for it. We are continuously bringing through creativity from Source and manifesting it into the physical. Then, we mostly use rational, logical systems created by someone's brain years ago, to reveal this creativity to the world. We have always wanted to share this creativity, and yet we have internalised fear-based controls to this natural flow.

**Rose:** One way we do this is through the old business paradigm?

**Donna:** Yes, we have many ideas every day. An idea captures our imagination and we want to materialise it and share it. In the old paradigm, we force ourselves to make money, play the game and feel worthy. When we build a business, we create a strategy for the business; including a five year plan; a marketing plan on how to "make" the world see it; a vision, usually with our idea strangled by large hairy growth goals; an operations plan: who, how and where; timelines to "make it happen" within certain times. We take on lawyers, accountants, marketers, to create rational, logical relationships for us. We usually open bank accounts with money we don't have and begin to create debt. We spend hours, money and time, dodging the tax system, and yet we are part of that system because we signed up to it by forming an entity. We copyright and patent everything so that no one will steal our idea. We often struggle and stress alone to "make all this happen." We often pay huge amounts of money we don't have, to "make all this happen." We often inspire others to come on board and lead the way to "make all this happen."

More often than not, our idea, that pure, beautiful piece of creativity is lost. It's lost to conflict, stress, lack, fatigue, loss, no time with friends and family, and no time with self. What was that beautiful pure piece of creativity again? What happened to the fine idea that inspired me in the beginning and made my heart sing? This story is one based on fear. We have business schools, universities, coaches, facilitators, online systems; all teaching us this old paradigm. We defend it, hold onto it, create new words and processes that look and sound better, but it's still the same fear-based system created to control us.

## A time of transformation

We are in a time of huge transformation in our evolutionary process and no one person has the answers for our next evolution, our next paradigm shift. It's an extremely challenging time, as we have learned so much about the old paradigm, and it seems to have worked for many. Through all our co-creative projects, I am feeling in this time of transformation, we are being challenged alone and together, to go beyond our knowledge, experience, teaching and dreams, and we are being dared to take a leap of trust.

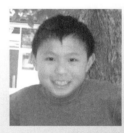

*Ray: A Sweet Seed*

*If I was to plant a WHOLE NEW WORLD seed it would be a strawberry because strawberries are sweet and I want my world to be sweet without any wars anger envy or greed. I would still want the blue sky, trees and clouds but no industrial or unnatural things like cars or hydraulic excavators. There won't be any pollution. My world would have people who are kind helpful and positive in everything. We will be running free and learning and teaching every day. There would be animals running free in the grass and in woods. We would still eat and kill them but we won't waste any.*

**Rose**: What would that leap of trust be? How do you see an alternative to "making things happen"? Can you give an example of how this works in one of your co-creative projects?

**Donna:** Open Arted, is an experimental co-creating community bringing together many skills, talents, knowledge, gifts, and ways of knowing. A group of talented artists heard the call to come together and plant a seed of co-creation. No entity, structure, or process has been put in place. The whole project is based on trust, great love, willingness to experiment, go with the flow, and provide mutual support and resources.

The artists create and are encouraged and supported to fully express themselves. Together with a service team of two, they are learning to co-create a regular monthly income, with each artist contributing from sales of their work. It's an amazing experiment in that each person is responsible for his or her own taxes and expenses, and whatever income flows through the bank account each month, is shared equally, no matter who did what or who sold what! It's a huge shift from the old model, and very exciting.

**Rose:** It is indeed quite a radical shift for people to be willing to share their income in that way! Can you say a little about the process you engaged in to get there?

**Donna:** I have been experimenting and evolving my whole life, to find a way we can "live our passion", while serving the greater good. I have found through the choices I have made in my life, I am always in the right place at the right time, to experiment with something daring and new. Or is it really old and ancient? The process I have engaged in has been to fully explore the possibilities that come through to me and if it isn't fun, I have tended to leave it behind. In its simplest form, I ask the question: "What would love do?" That's it, Rose, as simple and difficult as that!

**Rose:** Another very exciting community project you are setting up is, "The Great New Zealand Street Party". Please say a little about the ideas behind this project, what support you have for the idea, and how it will work?

**Donna:** Yes, this is a very exciting co-creative project. "The Great New Zealand Street Party: Connecting our Nation". Imagine across New Zealand, on the same day, at the same time, people coming together to celebrate all that we are and all that we have, in the way of simple, diverse, unique street parties. Neighbours will be connecting and co-creating an opportunity to be together in a fun, safe and all inclusive way. People love street parties and the simplicity of a street party means that no matter what religion, culture, belief, race, colour, gender, or agenda you hold, all can take part.

There is no corporate sponsorship, no branding, no leader, no committee, nor not-for-profit running this event. The power is in the hands of the people! We have been in contact with all the mayoral offices up and down this beautiful country and the idea has been embraced and supported. A group of seed planters are joining together in mutual support and giving the resources of their time, energy, ideas and voice, to get the word out to New Zealand, to be ready, this country is about to connect at the grassroots!

# Robin Allison
## Building a flourishing world

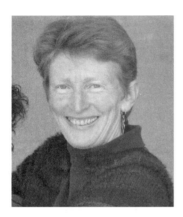

Robin is an architect and the founder and project co-ordinator of Earthsong Eco-Neighbourhood in Ranui, Waitakere City, which is a living demonstration of the principles of co-housing, permaculture and eco-architecture, and how they lead to social and environmental sustainability. Formerly with a practice in sustainable architecture, she is now moving more into consulting and speaking on sustainability issues, and is getting excited about being involved in an environmentally sustainable commercial redevelopment of her local suburban town centre. **www.earthsong.org.nz**

**Rose**: In thinking about living your passion, Robin, I imagine the main thing you'll want to talk about is Earthsong, which I've heard you describe as your soul work.

**Robin**: Well, Earthsong is the jewel at the centre of my life. Years ago, after many years of social awareness and environmental awareness I decided, this one life I have is possibly all I will ever have, and the world really needs us to be as aware, as connected and as intentional as possible. I decided to live in a way, to do as well as I can with this one incredibly privileged life I've been given. For me, that has meant nothing actually matters except making sure this planet's going to survive. Instead of running away from it all and going to live on a Green Peace boat, which I contemplated at one point and which was my first response, when I thought about it, I decided no, I have training in architecture, that's my skill and interest base. The most useful thing

I can do is to use the skills and training I have, and who I am in my situation in the world, and do it in a way that's the most effective use of my situation, rather than trying to join someone else's solution; and that's what I've been doing ever since.

I was drawn to architecture originally because it's in my family and I'm a visual person and quite creative. I'm also good at maths, physics and practical things. Architecture seemed to be the most useful skill using a whole lot of threads. Then too, I wanted a skill that would be effective in an alternative lifestyle; I was particularly interested in using alternative energy and solar energy. It's been a journey from there really.

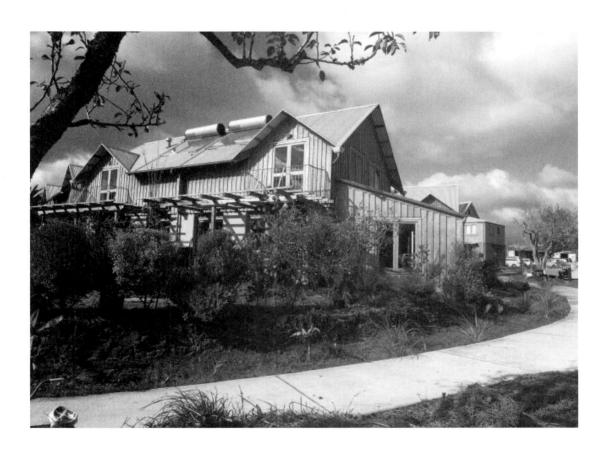

## *From vision to actuality*

**Rose**: Did you have a vision for Earthsong and has it evolved?

**Robin**: It's evolved since 1989. I'd completed my degree, had two little children and was at the very beginning of my career, struggling a bit with mainstream architecture and where I fitted with it. That's when I found a co-housing book and it was one of those ah-ha moments. Yes, I want to live in this sort of community with all these social and environmental aspects! Co-housing is self-created community by people who want to live in a more co-operative world. Co-housing itself is about social organization; a group of people get together, talk about how they really want to live, then they start the whole process and develop housing, which is designed for intentional community, but also has safety and privacy. To that co-housing model, I also added the other half of it for me: the environmentally sustainable building, design, energy, and all of that. I guess I found the book in 1989. Then there was a group in the early 90's, which I was part of for three years, looking at finding land outside Auckland. When that vision faded in late '94, I finally acknowledged nothing was going to eventuate from that group and realistically I much preferred to stay in the city. I'm a city sort of person and my kids were coming up to the teenage years. Actually, I think it's more important to find a way to live more sustainably in cities than in rural areas; we need those solutions rather than building ever more houses in rural areas. So I refocused my attention on an urban or suburban community, based on co-housing principles, permaculture and sustainable building.

**Rose**: Is Earthsong the only one of its kind?

**Robin**: It is, and the key came from redefining what it was I really wanted to do. I was still wondering where were all the other people who wanted to do it as well and then at Heart Politics, I talked about this at the sharing circle, and Warwick Pudney and Katrina Shields came up to me and said they'd support me to get it started. They said: "Look, you actually don't need anyone else at this stage. You need to clarify and write down your vision and people will either come or they won't." That was really very helpful and I realized I didn't need to wait until there were other people involved. Yet since then, it has been very much a jointly carried vision; people have been drawn in by that vision and carried it on their own.

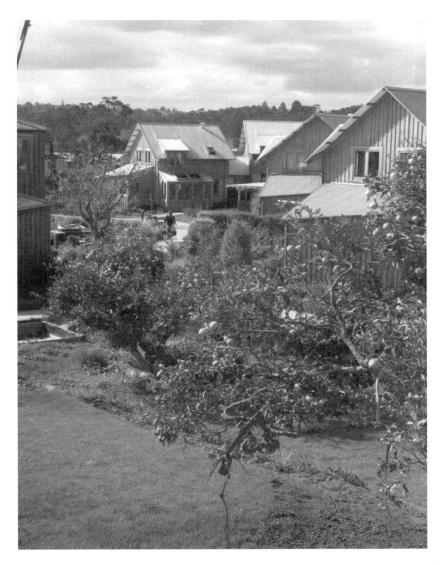

**Rose**: Did you spend much time creating the vision in detail?

**Robin**: In terms of the actual written words, our vision statement is almost identical to the one that evolved during the co-village group phase. I changed it to co-housing, permaculture, and so on, but really it evolved out of that initial group. When a lot of people joined the Earthsong project, we expanded it into three little subsections, which were written by those early founders. It's been that way since '95 now.

We haven't changed it. We've been back, looked and said: "That's good, we like it, and we want to keep going with that."

**Rose**: It seems, when there's a clear vision, it carries the project.

**Robin**: Yes, I learned a lot from that eco-village period, those first years. For instance, it sucks a lot of energy from the project, if new people arrive and want to revisit things we've already spent a lot of time talking about and decided upon. Therefore, right at the beginning, I was clear I didn't want to go back and renegotiate whether it was a rural or suburban project. I came to the point of being able to say: "No actually, this is what the project is. If you want to join that's fantastic, you can be fully part of developing it. If you want to revisit some of those things, please go and do your own project!" That clarity has been really important to ensure we continually move forward rather than be dragged back to things already decided.

**Rose:** You're clearly holding the boundaries!

**Robin**: Absolutely. There's nothing to stop someone else having a slightly different vision and going for it themselves, but we don't need to be diverted to accommodate every new person that comes along. Yet if new people do come with something that catches the energy of the group sufficiently, if half the people want to revisit it, we're still open to that. It's not that we're fixed and rigid and can never change. We're not going to change for one or two people, but we'll look at it, if there's real energy in the group to do so.

**Rose**: When you say "we" are you talking about a core group?

**Robin**: I'm talking about "we", the whole group, which at the moment consists of thirty-one households. There's probably a whole heap more who have been members and then there's a whole lot of renters at Earthsong as well, who are part of the decision-making. It's hard to put a fixed number on it.

**Rose**: You don't have to be a resident to be a member?

**Robin**: No and you don't have to be an owner. You have to be a member of Earthsong and that's a specific process. There are probably fifty or sixty active members.

**Rose**: What's been the most challenging, managing the building project or working with the people? I imagine they both have their own challenges.

**Robin**: They certainly do. It's been a very, very long journey. We've had major interpersonal challenges and major building challenges too. There've certainly been some tough times in both areas and some really good things as well.

**Rose**: At the end of fifteen years, do you still feel just as passionate about Earthsong?

**Robin**: Yes, it's great! It's a really great place to live and it feels completely congruent with what I imagined. As it has turned out, there's nothing that feels really different from the way we envisaged, although certainly things have taken a different direction. Part of being a group is accepting that things will take a slightly different direction than any individual might want. The whole is greater than any one part.

## *Becoming a servant leader*

**Rose:** It's a co-creative process, yet at the same time, you've been central to it?

**Robin**: Basically, yes. It's only quite recently I've been able to acknowledge that. It's a tough area and there's a real tension between these two things. I don't think it could have happened without a really empowered group, people who felt an equal responsibility to take part. I don't think such a group could develop a construction project, although it might work in an organisational context. Having an empowered co-creative group alongside a project leader is not a situation we're very familiar with. It's not the way things happen here. Usually there's a committee with a leader and followers, or there's an equal group. Yes, there's definitely a tension there. I guess I try to play down to what extent it might have been reliant on me, because that gets people's backs up.

**Rose:** Did you see yourself as a visionary leader before you started, or is that something you grew into?

**Robin**: No, I'm a quiet, shy introvert by nature, so it's very surprising to me. I don't see myself as a leader particularly, but I think that's helped the whole balance between leadership and the group.

**Rose**: If you'd been more extrovert and full-on, people might have reacted against you more?

**Robin**: Absolutely.

**Rose**: It does sound a tricky thing, this line between group process and leadership.

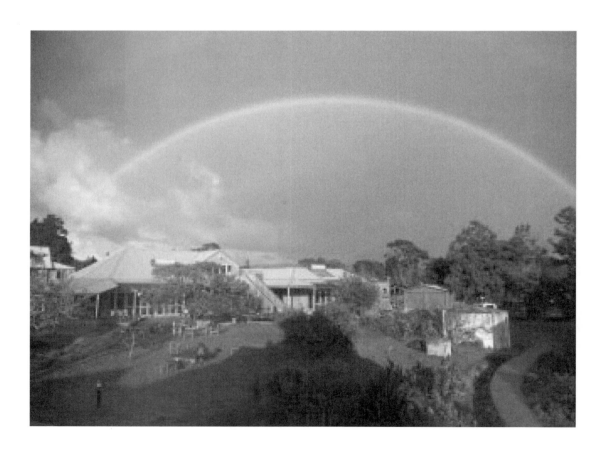

**Robin**: It is and I feel at times my motives have been misinterpreted, because people come with their own stuff about authority figures. We've had some battles which I thought were not generated by me and were quite unfair, but we're all on our own journeys and at different stages, so it probably goes with the territory. It's certainly one of the more painful sides of it.

**Rose**: It's a real service you've been doing.

**Robin**: It is! It's actually my spiritual practice. It feels like the way I can be of most service to the planet. About eight years ago, I made a whole shift to dedicating my life to Gaia. That's the most important thing: that I do whatever the planet needs to keep healthy.

**Rose**: It's a real soul commitment.

**Robin**: Yes!

**Rose**: Within all that, can you identify some of the most important skills you've developed to manage it all? I'm thinking in terms of managing people, the organisational side. I know for me a spiritual practice means I have certain ways to manage myself in order to maintain my priorities.

**Robin:** One of the things that's been really important is, I've had to keep strong boundaries between me and my job, myself and my neighbour. In order to survive as a human being, I've had to put boundaries around my work life in terms of when I'm available to people; otherwise, with living, working and being neighbours to the same people who are employing me, there'd be no me left! That puts a bit of difference between me and other people. For me, the most important thing was getting Earthsong built and that took precedence over being chummy and neighbourly. A few times incidents arose where I was friends with people and then, they wanted something to which I had to say no, so it became a personal thing, rather than a job thing. I found it hard to keep both types of relationships going with the same people. It became clear to me the whole of Earthsong is my priority, not individual relationships. This has been hard! It's kept me a bit separate and unsupported too. But there's a shifting now, which is really nice.

**Rose:** I've been wondering where you've found your support. To what extent have Heart Politics and the Tauhara wananga been helpful?

**Robin:** Fantastically so! Actually they've been the most helpful! They have been my support group. They kept me going! Just being with a group of people for four or five days, people who are peers, with whom I have a peer relationship, is so refreshing!

**Rose:** You can go there and shed your roles?

**Robin**: Yes and be a big person without fearing somebody might think I'm too big; a big person amongst big people.

**Rose**: They've been following your journey and cheering you on?

**Robin**: It's been great, and it's also kept me honest and accountable. I've known I'll go back to the group twice a year and say: "This is what happened this time and this is how I dealt with it"; knowing in my Earthsong life, I want to do things totally transparently and in total integrity, because I'm accountable to this other group, Heart Politics. Supported by, and accountable to; it always helps to have a little spur like that so you don't get complacent.

**Rose:** Have you been regularly to Heart Politics?

**Robin**: I go twice a year. I've been a trustee for quite a few years now. It's been very important to me; I've had a service role there also.

**Rose:** One aspect emerging for me out of this conversation is the theme of servant leadership. This appears to be the role you've stepped into, not knowing that's what you were doing at the beginning.

**Robin:** I certainly didn't have that concept, but that's always been how it's felt, yes. I've never done any of it for my personal power and fame, which is sometimes how other people might interpret it.

**Rose:** There's nothing wrong with liking to be acknowledged and having what you've created admired. It's natural, really.

**Robin:** In lots of small ways, yes of course, I get a kick out of people saying how wonderful it is, but that's certainly not the motivation for doing it.

**Rose:** So clarity, strength of vision, and the willingness to put yourself in service to the vision, seem to be central to the success of this project. Is there anything else you'd like to add, to sum up?

**Robin:** I feel it's important for each person to look at their own life, what they have control over and the sorts of choices they do have, and to live as consciously as possible, knowing that none of us can exist without a flourishing world. If the world's not flourishing, it diminishes the extent to which any of us, as individuals, can flourish. I have an incredibly full and rich life now. The more you give out, the more you get back. I'm not flourishing in the financial sense, but my life feels very full and abundant. That's the most important thing. We could talk about sustainability ad infinitum. To sustain is a good thing, we need to do that, but really it's only the very first basic level. Actually flourishing is what I'm interested in now. Let's create a flourishing world!

# Margaret Jefferies
## Getting in the groove

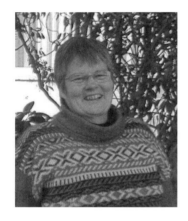

Community work has been in my life always. Initially I trained as a post primary teacher, but becoming a mother of five children (two sets of twins and one daughter with Down Syndrome) I was daily involved with others in the community. When the bulk of my family's needs were over, I became more involved with the community. My parents always believed I could do anything. I was loved. This is a tremendous heritage to have, so from this I have a strong belief that anything is possible and I can take on whatever I am drawn to. Currently I am chair of Project Port Lyttelton and in that role touch many of its various projects. My strong points are an ability to inspire people, bring them together and let them see their abilities; networking; thinking globally and acting locally; holding an intention and holding the values of a group. I'm good at dreaming up ideas and seizing opportunities. I like to have fun and I laugh a lot. I have a Masters degree and diplomas in music, teaching and theology. www.lyttelton. net.nz

**Rose:** What does it mean to you to live your passion, Margaret?

**Margaret:** The creative spirit is relentless and it keeps on going! As soon as something's created, you don't sit back, relax and say wow, the next thing comes on! I'm allowing myself to do what touches my heart, to be bold and to ask questions. It's part of our mission statement to make Lyttelton, a sustainable vibrant town, and one of the skills I bring to the whole thing, is a focus on the core values, making sure we're touching base with those values continually.

There are several things that come in behind me to do this. One is the state of where we are on the Earth and the urgency of that. The fact that I'm sixty-two, I know I can't muck around and say I'll do this next year, I've got to do it now! The other thing is the momentum is so strong now, it's an evolving thing. I think back to when I was about fifty and was asking: "What am I going to do ten years from now?" I listed all the things I was good at and worked out how I could do them. This led to something, and from there to organising the Spirit at Work conferences. While I was doing this, I was growing at a personal level and was evolving what I would like for this country and I started speaking out about that. After doing those three conferences on spirituality in the workplace, I asked myself what was *my* workplace? My answer was my community, so that became my challenge!

*Adam Matthew earning Time Bank credits.*

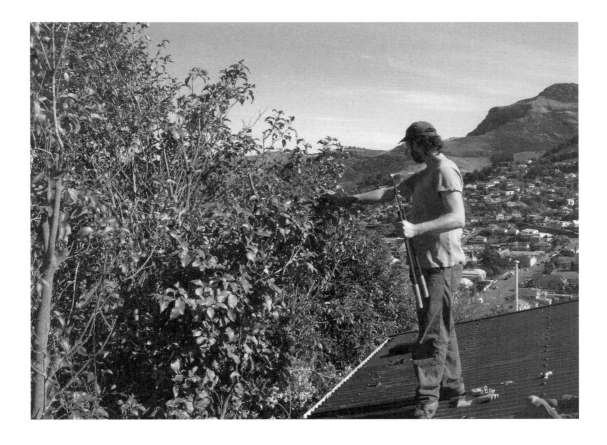

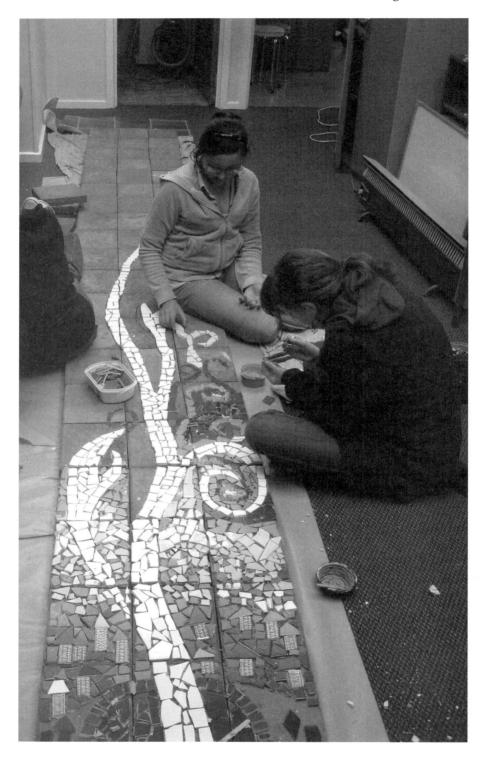

We called as many people as we could together and co-created a mission statement. We used that as a measure for what to take on board. Sustainability was the key word, but it's a bit like action research, you move towards something, and then something else comes up in the process. It's co-creative. It's not as though I have a sterile blueprint. The ideas are all there, but the unfolding can be a little bit different as time goes by. As the novelists say, the characters take over!

It feels to me one of my chief roles is to hold the values. I watch Wendy who's younger and has a lot of energy and no way could I do the things she's doing. I do a lot of physical jobs as well, but my main one is holding that space, holding that stake in the ground, reminding people as they say things, to check those values out first.

**Rose:** That's so important. I think there's something about our age group, people in their fifties and sixties, wanting to give back the fruits of their experience and wisdom. I know you and Wendy are making a profound difference in Lyttelton. You've developed a group of at least forty volunteers; you've set up a farmer's market, a waste minimisation scheme, and summer and winter festivals.

**Margaret:** Yes, and we have a community garden, which hopefully at some stage, may feed into the farmer's market. We're actually making quite a difference economically to the town. On Saturday you can't find a parking space anywhere and all the cafes are full with people coming out to the market. We have a community building we're renovating and the top floor is functioning well now; that's where we have our office. The floor down below will be a community art space, where everyone in the community can have access and play with art. We have a community van in which we take people who find transport a challenge, to their appointments and shopping. There's a time bank and I'm really excited now, because although it's taken a couple of years, we've got a time broker and funding from the Tindall Foundation. We've also managed to get sponsorship trialling software, so people can do time banking by phone or directly on the Internet. We're developing our website and that's looking good. We print a newspaper, Lyttelton News, and in that I try to come from an appreciative inquiry point of view. I like to hear the stories and I do a lot of interviews with

*Community art, making mosaics for the Festival of Lights.*

people. There's definitely been a shift to a more positive energy. I heard back from a school secretary who's been here for years; a lady who's well on into her 80's and another woman who works at the hotel bar, all old time Lyttelton people who are appreciating what we're doing.

**Rose:** I believe the project is becoming a catalyst to bring other groups together? That's very exciting!

## Bigger conversations and new alliances

**Margaret:** Project Port Lyttelton is just one group in Lyttelton. You have other groups, like Lions, Rotary, the Business Association, Information Centre and the Residents Group. A number of us have been talking and saying it's silly reinventing the wheel and duplicating things. We're only three thousand people, why not work together more as a group? The Business Association, Project Port Lyttelton and the Information Centre are all thinking, "Yes, let's start doing things together". I heard Bliss Browne of "Imagine Chicago" is going to be in New Zealand at the end of May, so I've been talking to her, and she's willing to come here, and we're thinking, not just Lyttelton but the whole harbour basin! We're starting to get a name in the City as those who trial new models of social cooperativeness. Wendy's been talking to the Ministry of Social Development and they're always looking for grassroots examples that are going well. I went to a meeting with seven or eight overseas experts in Christchurch last week and it was so encouraging to hear them talking about sustainability. Both Wendy and I were there and we felt good being able to say: "We're doing all this!" It was affirming. The discussion was about play, celebration, embedded leadership, not top down.

**Rose:** That's all out there in the mainstream? Policy makers are starting to consider these important concepts?

**Margaret:** It was interesting, because it was held at the University and when it was question time I stood up, and the question was not really for the panel; it was more a challenge to the University: "We want to have a relationship with you as partners. You can help with research and we can be the on-the-ground people". That sort of partnering happens a lot in Murdoch University, Western Australia and has been very successful, but it doesn't happen here at Canterbury yet. I hope it will.

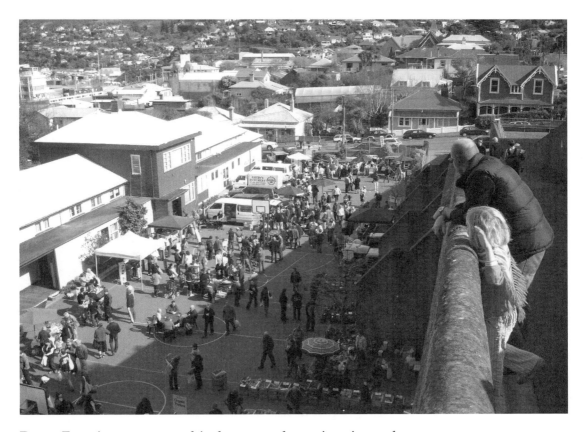

**Rose:** Forming a partnership between the university and your grass-roots project would extend the co-creative community even more, bringing the head and the heart together. It sounds as if it's all developing beyond your wildest dreams?

*The Farmers' Market*

## Thinking as a community

**Margaret:** I actually say, you could call it spiritual, but if you don't want to use that term, you could call it being in the groove. You know, when jazz or other musicians play together, they get in the groove and that's when things fly. You're playing along, when suddenly you're in the groove, and everything's just going, not smoothly, but beautifully. I think that's what I'm waiting for; the moment we actually perform as a community, as a whole community, not as a lot of people within the community.

It's really like creating a self-fulfilling prophecy, telling people how good they are. That's when they move towards it.

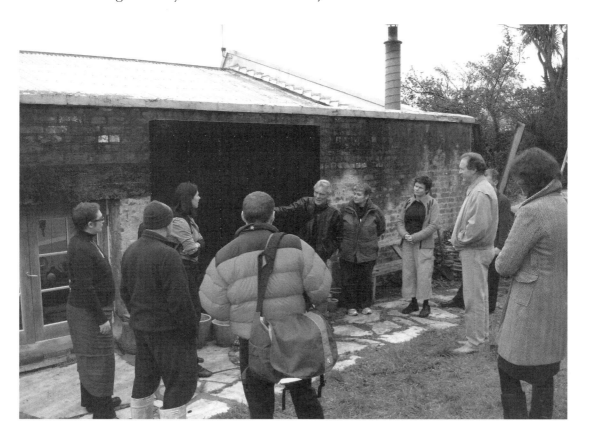

*Jayashri and the warm wall.*

## *Postscript:*

Sadly, not long after our interview, Margaret had a fall whilst at a conference in Australia and was diagnosed with a heart problem. Continuing with unfailing commitment and optimism, Margaret sent me this update on how others have stepped in to keep the community "in the groove".

I was talking about community coming together, as it were, in the groove. Well today, I am delighted to see that happening. Since I had a fall in Australia, resulting in having a heart problem diagnosed, I have drawn back a little from the physical work and I've been amazed at what's happening. People are stepping into the gaps! There's a young woman, Helene Smith who, I tell people, is an upcoming leader in this community. She told me today, I say this to her so much, she is beginning to believe it. Well, today she talked about what she is doing, and it's magic! She's facilitating this in "the groove stuff" I 'm talking about. She's linking with so many people, and linking them with each other, and getting them involved in creative ways. I am astounded. It's so beautiful to watch.

Another person, Tiri Pharazyn, has come to join Chris Twemlow in doing the Time Bank. She is another weaver of magic! She's so in love with each person she meets in the community that her excitement rubs off on everyone. She is engaging people in the Time Bank concept and they are responding. I know she feels blessed to have found this job, as it is the sort of thing she has dreamed of doing, pulling people together within a community so that each person's needs are met.

A new development happening here came from a proposal to CPIT (Christchurch's polytechnic) for the use of their Seven Oaks organic site: two acres, rent free for three years, on which we will start a business growing organic produce for the community. Our proposal has been accepted, so now a new adventure unfolds! With this, and the farmer's market, we can generate an income for the community. This means we can develop the projects we want without having to get approval from a funding body. We are having a working bee on Sunday to clear some of the land. I put out for volunteers and already four people, who I don't even know, are coming!

There is a spirit of aliveness, a juiciness, an amazement at what can be achieved in this town. It is infectious!

# *James Samuel*
## Making a gentle footprint as we handle the basics

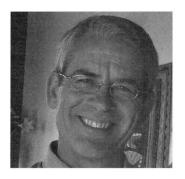

I was born in England and did most of my growing up in New Zealand. I left home at sixteen and found myself at the Findhorn Community in 1977, aged twenty. From there, I joined a spiritual community as a follower of Bubba Free John, as he was at the time. This became my path for fifteen years. It was a really full intensive life of service, karma yoga and meditation. From the age of twenty-three to thirty-eight, I wasn't at all aware of what was happening in the world around me, so just prior to my fortieth birthday, I started a new journey of exploration discovering the world I was living in and was able to look at political and environmental crises from a spiritual perspective. I had moved to Waiheke Island and as I became involved in the community, there was a slow progression from wanting to understand the world better, to creating a blog, showing documentary films, facilitating dialogue circles and joining co-creators. Then last year my partner Kim and I had a beautiful baby, Zuva, and a whole new life began! Blog: www.yesterdaysfuture.net

**James:** There's a practice and a test involved in living my passion. I have a practice of living in trust. It's something I came to a number of years ago when I looked at what my values were. Trust is the thing I value most. It's about trusting that if I have something to contribute, my needs will be met. How that actually plays out is an interesting one; there are times when trust is tested. The doubting mind kicks in and starts to question: "What are you going to do now? You don't have anywhere to live next week, or how are you going to pay the bills? Maybe I should just go and get a regular job?"

My passion is also fed by some clarity I came to a few years back about what I did and didn't want. That's what got me to Waiheke Island. I became very clear I wanted to contribute to community using the skills I have. I wanted to live somewhere where there was clean air, clean water, healthy, happy people making conscious, intelligent choices about their lives and their relationship to their environment, and to serve that community with my own skills, talents and experience. When I got clear about all of that, two days later a friend I hadn't heard from for years emailed me and said: "I've just bought an eight acre organic orchard on Waiheke, would you like to come and join me?"

I guess part of my passion is also fed by what I have learned about the world and how it seems to work and function. That came about from two or three years of fairly intensive research into areas of life I hadn't previously known. I'd been cloistered away in a spiritual community for fifteen years and hadn't read the papers, watched tv, or listened to the radio. I had no idea what the power structures were or what was happening to our environment. I wanted to dig deeper and find out. I feel incredibly grateful for that time of exploration because I was able to look at the things I was discovering about the world, such as the environmental crisis and the geo-political dramas that were playing out, from a spiritual perspective. Although I am a remarkably detailed person, I was able to look at them

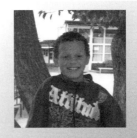

*Andre: A Money Seed*

My WHOLE NEW WORLD seed would be an everlasting money tree and it will grow into a world where all the countries are joined together so everyone can take from the tree for food water and shelter.

from a really big overview, to have a global and greater-than-Earth view of what these manifestations are. I was asking, why is this manifesting and what human characteristics, qualities and emotions are playing out here? What is this as a spiritual process? Those years were most helpful. They allowed me to explore my dark side and this in turn, was an exploration of the dark side of the world and how one affects the other. It's absurd to point the finger at an individual, as many of us love to do. Political figures are simply representing qualities in ourselves which we prefer not to look at. Until we each confront those aspects of ourselves, these manifestations will continue.

I have a very strong sense that the current form of society as it's promoted on tv is not sustainable. It's in deep trouble and that's reflected in all kinds of dysfunctions in society and communities. My interest is to support people to find ways to come to a greater place of trust with each other. Part of that involves all the practical things that relate to food, shelter and clothing, because if we handle those basics, then all sorts of other wonderful creative possibilities exist for us to explore also. We can meet those needs in a way that is very, very gentle on our environment and creates a very gentle footprint.

**Rose:** I'm hearing there are two realities. One is the reality you've discovered, which is based on trust and reciprocity, in which you put something out and something comes back to take care of you. The other reality is the world in trouble.

**James:** For a couple of years my passion was disseminating information, sharing information about the state of the world and the things I was discovering. That's what I did through blogs and through the making of documentary film and later on, the finding and screening of documentary film. In December last year, I realized this is a new moment and I felt like I'd learned enough about how the world works. You can keep learning and finding more and more detail forever and ever. The fact there were a few pieces missing didn't really matter, I could see the whole picture and felt I didn't need to focus there anymore. What we really need are examples of how to create something different, so I started looking at that. As soon as I put my attention there, all kinds of other things began to come towards me, which was really amazing! Literally, as soon as I changed my focus of attention, all these solutions materialised and started coming forward. It was beautiful!

**Rose:** It's a powerful and empowering process when this happens.

**James:** Yeah! Where we put our attention is what we get!

# *A local/global vision for Waiheke Island*

**Rose:** What are you up to now?

**James:** Having a baby has changed my life quite a bit in the last months! I guess I'm learning to be more focused on the leverage points, because I don't have as much time to put into the details. A lot of it's about conversations, networking and connecting people who are coming forward from all kinds of different places. It's about building relationships of trust and seeing what grows out of that.

Documentary film is probably one of the most effective forms of communication there is, where you can actually learn quite a complex subject in a very compressed time frame. Whereas, to gain that information through reading, would take a book or two. I enjoy the process of watching a film and having a dialogue circle afterwards. It's a really powerful way of grounding information and making it very real for people, because they can express their own feelings about something. They have the opportunity to listen to other views, and have others inform their views. The dialogue tools are something I really appreciate and enjoy immensely. Last year I facilitated dialogue circles with a group of people to see what we could do about furthering local self government on the island. If there's one thing that focuses my energy, it's this thing of localisation: meeting our needs and making our decisions locally, self government, local food production, information sharing, dialogue, creative housing/shelter solutions, and creative uses of land. This is not self sufficiency in some kind of exclusive way that cuts us off from other communities. The Internet is beautiful in that it allows us to connect communities globally, so we can learn from each other.

It's so important to hold a space for people to start to trust each other and to be creative in how we learn to identify and meet our needs. It seems, when we're not living in trust, then that's when we become exaggerated, wanting to build great empires and fortunes, acquire lots of money and property, and put up fences. It's all done out of fear. There's a real wave of people starting to wake up now and realize that actually, we're all in this together. We can have fun with this. It's actually not that hard.

**Rose:** We need dialogue circles to augment a sense of oneness and acceptance of differences, taking the conversation into a deeper or higher place, don't we?

**James:** Yes, and to allow different points of view to be expressed. We see things through filters that can end up filtering out something that's really valuable. We may assume that what a person says fits in a box in our mind, but if we can get beyond our prejudices and preconceptions and really hear each other, we'll probably find there are all sorts of creative possibilities and solutions.

**Rose:** I believe the sense of oneness, being part of a bigger family, comes from expressing all of who we are, rather than making ourselves smaller to fit in. That's what comes from dialogue for me: to be able to

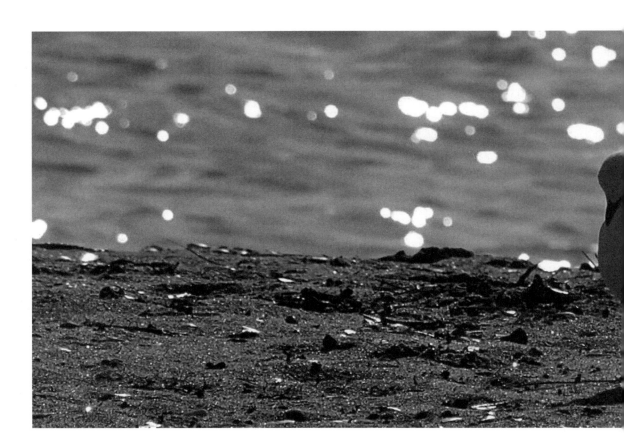

embrace all of each person is a stretch, but that's what we need to do to become more interconnected and inclusive. Unconditional acceptance builds a container in which creativity can cook.

I like your vision of empowering local communities to be more self organizing. I guess Waiheke lends itself to such a vision because it's a relatively small island community which seems to attract people who are more alternative thinkers?

**James:** Yes, and having the natural geographical boundary of the coast means we can measure the inputs and outputs when we get to that stage. We're not there yet. A number of people feel Waiheke has an amazing opportunity, and an obligation, to demonstrate this self reliance and how we can take care of ourselves and the land on which we live. If we can't do it here, there's not much hope for the world! We're not doing it here yet and that's what I want to see. I want to see the island humming with all of these amazing creative initiatives popping

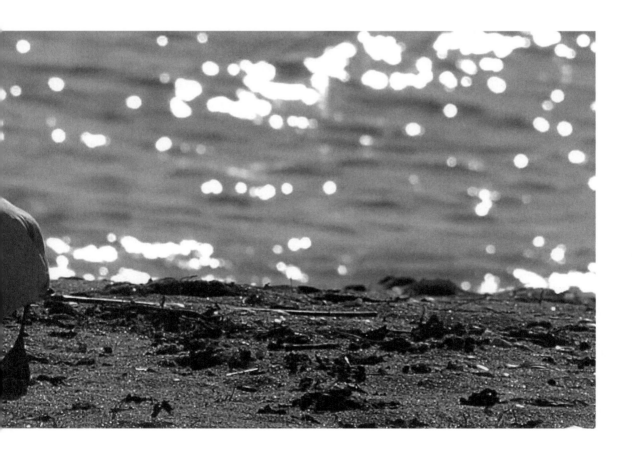

up all over and linked to each other, so that people aren't working independently and doubling up on their resources to achieve their ends. People are asking what we can do. Well, we can do lots if we work together. Individually we can do hardly anything at all, but we're powerful if we connect.

I've started talking with people from different groups on the island. We have a wananga where we can hear of each other's activities and needs, to see how we can work together a little more. We don't assume we're immediately going to bond, because it doesn't work like that. Natural little groups spring up, but if we can find ways to link them into a web so nobody feels isolated, that's got to be very powerful. Will and I are looking at a business hub to support community initiatives, using the yurt Kim and I have. We'll set it up, fill it with Hi-Tech IT gear, couches and art, and have a business hub that generates significant funds to support and hold the space for lots of these community initiatives.

The energy tends to get dissipated if there isn't some place for people to come together to connect on these projects, to witness the growth of them and be able to plug into them when they can. Here are all these different projects: we've got a notice board with pictures of the progress of a project, a description about it, who's involved, what's current, what's happening. With all these different initiatives, people can go: "I'm interested in that." or "I've got a few hours next week, do you need any help with that?" They don't need to know everything that preceded it, but they can get a sense of it. They don't need to know what's going to follow it, but they know somebody's holding a space for this, so if they put energy into it, it won't be wasted. Then people can just go: "Great I've got an afternoon. I'll put my energy into that!" I have a feeling things will progress fast if that space is held!

**Rose:** It sounds like building an attractor field of people's combined energies, similar to what's happening with the Co-Creators group, but on an island-wide scale. All sorts of new things can emerge from those meetings.

**James:** Lots of connections can be made between people, as well as having that physical space and those physical representations, if we have the IT support, we can also network people online as well. Then, for example, the online facilitation course I'm doing can be used to facilitate those processes. Will's talking about a Waiheke portal people can plug into: click that link and go to the Waiheke portal. You've got current news; what's happening; a calendar of events. Then you can go from there into various forums and discussions about things that are going on. There's a lot of clued up people, who won't necessarily come out of their houses very often to get involved in things, but if they're there and they have things to contribute, and if they get excited enough, they'll get involved. There are a lot of resources: a lot of money, wisdom, skill and experience. By having a physical place as well as an online place, people can connect. Then I think we've got something to really build on and grow! Everything from food growing: put your order in for your food. For really organized car sharing, click here: if you need a car at such and such a street, just pick it up there.

**Rose:** I'm hearing it's the communication and networking that excite you most, linking people, bringing people together, creating forums where sharing and co-creativity can happen and different views can be expressed and heard.

**James:** I tend to be a starter. I started the community garden and the food exchange which are going quite well. It's a really nice focal point and it makes people think; they're really delighted they can send along excess produce from their gardens in exchange for other produce. Or sometimes people come along and buy food, throw a few coins in, and that goes back to the community garden. It's a very simple gesture, but yeah, the facilitation thing, that's exciting!

# *Robina McCurdy*
## Listen to spirit and follow the synergy

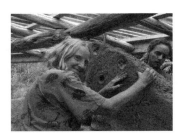

Robina is a 'sustainability catalyst'. All her life she has been involved in community educational initiatives and establishing practical demonstration models of sustainable systems. For three decades, she has been engaged in broad scale community development and, for the past twenty years, in permaculture design and teaching, organic growing, the development of environmental education resources and the creation of participatory processes for decision-making and collective action. She has taught and applied these powerful community-building methods with households, neighbourhoods, schools, farms, eco-villages, and bioregions, in Aotearoa/New Zealand, Australia, South Africa, Brazil, Ireland, Scotland, England, Canada and America. Robina's state and Steiner education training have provided her with the background to teach in many different contexts. Human capacity building is one of her special skills: inspiring, guiding and offering specific tools and techniques for people to access their gifts, develop their potential, build their resourcefulness and live their dreams. Robina founded two charitable trusts: Tui Land Trust (which includes Tui Community and is now renamed Tui Spiritual & Educational Trust) and the Institute of Earthcare Education Aotearoa. Much of her work is done through these organisations. **www.greenworld-earthcare.org**

**Robina:** Living my passion means not compromising what motivates me forward into action; what propels me to do what I do. My passion is social change, environmental restoration, and contributing energy to turn around a situation for the betterment of the whole. The inner feeds the outer and the outer feeds the inner. It's a complete cycle.

After working in service to Gaia and humanity for most of my life, at fifty-seven years of age, I am utilising my facilitation skills to achieve something which is for me and my partner, Huckleberry. My most recent project is the building of our own home! This has been continuing for most of the past two years. The principle behind it is deep sustainability. All the materials either come from the site, for example, the clay and sand, or from within our bioregion. In deciding what materials to use on the house, we take our thinking as far as possible, for low impact on the planet.

Earth-building as a technique, and earth as a material, really ask for hands-on labour intensity. In this case, our place is seven metres in diameter, plus an outdoor kitchen of a couple of metres diameter, that equates to maybe six or seven people working together. We chose not to make this an arduous project, slogging away for years on end by ourselves or hiring people, but a project which could train and empower, particularly young people, in the techniques of earth-building. So we turned this opportunity into an internship and apprenticeship. Everyone thought they were coming for earth-building. While we lived in the same rented house and associated caravans at Tui, having our own cook, a regular sharing circle in the morning, with developed support systems, venturing on wilderness and social adventures, we discovered we were strongly building community in a deep and spiritual way. Using virtually no power tools and doing almost all the work by hand made the experience a person to person, quiet, slow activity, building depth of relationship.

*Katy:*
*A Co-operation Seed*

*If I planted a Co-operation seed it would grow a new world that will work together to make things better. It would have light, blue, clean water with lots of colourful fish. Nice big buildings, lots of companies with joy and smiles on all faces. Lots of big green land and schools. All the stuff we make will work together.*

**Rose:** Very holistic.

**Robina:** Incredibly holistic in every way. When new people come and stay and want to have a go at building, they're people who are learning from us, while we're learning from professionals like Richard Walker, an earth-building architect in mud brick, mostly adobe, and Kreyn, his son, who builds in cob. We'll have them teach us a new technique for a few hours when we're at that stage and pay them their professional wages for that duration, then we'll work at it ourselves and learn new things, sharing and exploring with each other, then we'll come to the next stage. We do similarly for our interns, passing on those techniques, and very quickly they become teachers themselves. We're documenting all the technical side and all the stages of development photographically, and keeping a diary record and recipes, for example, of the sealing pastes and so on, so we're building a resource for other people doing something similar. In this way our learning is further passed on. That's how to make building your own home an educational experience and a service to others!

The other part of it is empowerment of people's creativity. For example, today we were trying to figure out how to adhere cob to glass, because we want to frame up a free standing glass window, so I've been adhering barbed wire onto it, just as an experiment. I said to one of the young people working with me today, "I want to have this kind of pattern or feeling in the mosaic that's on the wall" and she scribed it and threw a few things on paper with colour. I'll leave her totally to it, just give a little feedback every now and again, and she'll adjust what she's doing accordingly and execute it.

The house is really a resonance of around sixty people of all ages, but mostly, young people's creative energy and practicality. It reflects back to them and gives them the message: "I want to create my own home in a way that isn't just a house; rather it's a structure resonating with spirit, a spiritual sanctuary."

It's never been "just a building project". We'd go out to gather rocks, say for the kitchen stone wall and people chose rocks that pleased them. As part of that rock gathering, we also went for a swim in a swimming hole and connected with the source of rocks from the river, bringing people closer to knowing the Golden Bay geology. We had a chain gang of twenty people passing rocks up to build the wall, so we'd harvest the material, make a connection with the place it came from, and then use it in a transformed way.

I believe co-creative community needs a common project and a common philosophical focus. But more importantly, running through that project, is a service dimension, which is beyond the benefit of one individual or a commercial enterprise. Exploring a new edge of learning together will sustain the motivation.

**Rose**: I understand a co-creative community to be a group of people coming together to create something, and transcending the individualistic paradigm most of us have been brought up in, moving towards a sense of interconnectedness, interdependence, connection with nature as well: a holistic way of working together. I'm interested in identifying the factors that build a successful co-creative community. I'm imagining a group of young people, mostly in their twenties, coming together from different parts of the world. They land at Tui and they're there for several months. What do you, as the facilitator, put in place in order for it to work?

**Robina:** Firstly, people all need to pull together to manage the physical environment. In this case, that means managing the house we're living in, doing the chores, keeping the house clean, cooking and so on; self organising around that with a little bit of guidance, if necessary. The self organising is very important.

## A sharing circle

Another part is to have a scheduled regular time for a sharing circle once a week. If we weren't on a task-oriented project, with a certain amount of work to be accomplished, it would have been more regular. The focus is on: "How's it going for you? How are you doing? Anything you need to share with the whole group?" We start off with an attunement, to be still, to honour the land and the project, and to call in spirit in a simple way. Then the sharing circle has two parts, one is personal, and people sometimes talk about how it's going with their families back home and how that's affecting them, or they talk about what's coming up for them generally and in their relationships with each other. It's a deep feelings sharing and we pass around a "talking stone" to hold the focus. Each person is fully listened to, and for many of them this is the first time they've really been listened to. The next two rounds are about the practical aspects of the project. How is it going for each person? What are they learning? What would they like to be doing this week? Do they have any dissatisfaction? Then we finish with the plan for the coming week and any comments or questions. This generally takes half a morning, but we take as long as needed, given that we have practical work in mind too. This sharing circle is really, really important!

When conflict arises or differences need to be dealt with, I've learned it is very helpful to have a work-based trainer, or supervisor as my own mentor, somebody who is detached but also close and caring of our group to meet with weekly and bounce ideas off and trouble shoot with. I'd do this another time, for sure. It would also be great if each trainee also had their own local mentor, someone they could meet and share with, have a break from the group with, to get a refreshing reflection or new angle that person might bring in; maybe even have a meal together. A semi-parent figure or an auntie/uncle type figure, because people are often from overseas countries and everyone benefits from that kind of support.

Then there's balancing out the work focus, which can be pretty physically demanding, with leisure and doing things together that are really fun, such as musical evenings, educational presentations, saunas and special outings.

**Rose:** It's a transformational experience for everybody involved, including you. There's room for a lot of personal learning and healing and interpersonal learning as well as practical skills and communication.

**Robina:** Yes, another thing I did, and would have liked to have done more, and will definitely do with other groups, is to bring in various kinds of communication skills and personal tools. For example, participants didn't know how to deal with conflict or how to have strong enough boundaries to protect themselves spiritually, psychically and mentally from a person who commonly put people down, and was hurtful, and they asked for skills training in those areas. We did mini-workshops around the issues that pop up when you live in a co-creative community; so everyone can communicate skillfully and compassionately.

Many participants were at crossroads concerning the next steps in their lives, and for several this was whether to continue living in New Zealand and if so, how? I facilitated an individual goal setting mandala process with them for a morning and we shared together in a workshop. Out of that, every single person's goals have come to pass, very quickly. For example, four people who wanted New Zealand residency got it within six months, from a position of having no jobs and no prospects!

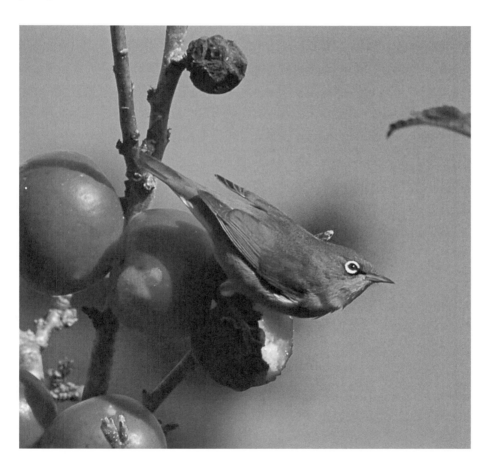

## *Manifesting from the flow of life*

**Rose:** What has been the greatest learning for you in this project? I imagine you must be learning all the time?

**Robina:** I guess broadly, there's a point at which every individual, then the collective of individuals, takes responsibility for the project, for their own learning, their own process, their own communication skills, and so on. You can actually pinpoint a moment, from one day to the next and stand back, just giving a little bit of guidance here and there, as well as bringing in resource materials, such as specific books, and then basically shift into an overseeing role watching the whole thing unfold. At this moment, if it's done from a place of non-ego attachment and service, a shift happens and another dimension emerges which is spirit led. I just look at the signs and feel the energy, listen to spirit and follow the synergy and the timing of everything. This quality of energy may shift my plans on a daily basis, even to what materials we need to build with that day.

What I've learned, and it's not a new learning but it's happened every single time without fail on this project, when I have needed, at each stage, another person with very specific skills, or another pair of hands, I visualize and ask for that very clearly with my mind's focus and look to the Universe for support and that person will show up the next day! For example, yesterday two women were working on the mosaic for the kitchen wall cob and I'd given them a bit too much freedom for their level of experience. They admitted, "We've mucked it up! We're actually out of our depth here!" And I said, "Well, it has to be complete. We can't give it any more time." They responded, "We really need help" and I replied, "let's then ask for it, here and now." That very afternoon, someone arrived at Tui with specific skills in mosaic on cob wall. He took over the project and completed it unsupervised by the evening! On another day I said, "Patrick, we really need another pair of hands. Please help me to put out to the Universe right now. Let's visualise and ask for another person to show up." Someone showed up that same night wanting to work on cob. Great! Another example: in Germany, they have a tradition of apprenticing in building, called the Journeyman. They move around and travel for two years or more, serving as builders to get diverse experience. They wear a distinctive outfit: a black hat and white shirt, black waistcoat and pants with braces. I needed someone to build, because I realized I didn't have the skills to create a really fine temporary composting toilet and it needed to be done that week. I only wanted someone for three days, then this Journeyman showed up three hours later and asked around, "Does anybody want any work done? I'm here for three days!" I said, "Oh, you must be the person I put the call out for!" This is the calibre of manifestation I'm experiencing!

**Rose:** There seem to be two things here: one is you create a container in which the group synergy can build. This container is made up of your common purpose, shared responsibility for the practical aspects of the project, timetable, guidelines, support processes, and so on. Then, you say, there's a moment when the process becomes spirit led, something happens at that moment, you notice what's happening and then step back?

**Robina:** With no interference. Give gentle guidance when needed, when it seems spirit is not flowing so strong, and reflect on what is the right thing for any given moment.

**Rose:** How do you know the moment has come?

**Robina:** On an energetic level, there's a harmony that comes in, a flow. People's energies are no longer bumping up against each other as personalities try to find a space. There's a relaxation in people's bodies. There's usually an increase in laughter, or song, or storytelling, or even concentrated mellow quietness. Those are some of the atmospheric indicators.

**Rose:** It's a shift in energy, an integration of some sort, a unifying. You're also talking about synchronicities, people showing up in response to your power of intention, the clarity of your focus. You visualise and you ask?

**Robina:** Yes, but it's not a long thing. I may do it for seconds only, then totally let it go, like breathing intention into a balloon as you blow it up, blessing it on its journey, then letting it go to the wind currents. I feel the calibre of response from spirit reflects the degree of service I am offering in this work.

**Rose:** I recognize what you're saying from my own experience in groups. It seems co-creative community is an energetic container which has a harmonic resonance to it, into which spirit can play and respond. A co-creation occurs between the group and spirit.

**Robina:** Absolutely! What I experienced in the building project is that this group of people recognized it. They said: "Something's going on here. What is it?" As we went deeper with it, they knew it. We didn't talk about it greatly or "wow" it, just accepted it as part of life when we are "moving in the wairua". Each of these people was drawn to the project; whether they were attracted to a building project in intentional community, knew of me or Huckleberry, went to our website, whatever; but every single person had their own kind of spiritual search and being here building with us was the outcome. Nobody was getting "out of it". There wasn't any escapism through drugs and alcohol. They were here to get "into it" fully, on a spiritual pursuit for a higher goal for themselves. I'm sure the combination of these particular people created the receptacle for spirit to dance!

**Rose:** It was a unity of intention?

**Robina:** Yes, even though each person came individually, unknown to the others and the spiritual aspect wasn't spelled out.

**Rose:** Great!

**Robina:** What's great is we're talking about a building project!

**Rose:** Some building project, Robina!

# TRANSFORMING BUSINESS

Transforming the way we do business to trade goods and services is fundamental to social change. Contemplating such changes causes us to question our relationship with money and what it means to be of service; aspects of life which offer great learning. Freeing the stuck energy of established patterns or forms, which are no longer serving their purpose, entails deconstructing the old forms, admitting at times we don't know the answers and being open to experiment with innovative ideas. True creativity arises through autonomous individuals and true autonomy recognizes an ethical responsibility to the whole. As more and more businesses now acknowledge, the greater whole includes employees, stake-holders, customers or clients, the environment, the local community and the global community.

Now, as the old ways of social organisation are breaking down, and the Earth is becoming less hospitable to our unwholesome practices, freedom to create new solutions which serve the good of all is not a luxury, but a necessity.

# *Shift Ten*

## From businesses which create huge profits for a few whilst destroying the environment, to new sustainable models of business which honour life and give back to communities.

The creative impulse to discover and invent new solutions to shared problems frequently involves freeing energy which has become stuck in established forms and opening to more inclusivity. Social entrepreneurs are developing new business models based on the principles of natural abundance, unity in diversity and community service.

# *Daniel Batten*
## Sensational serendipity

With no formal business training, in 2003, Daniel formed what has become a multimillion dollar high-tech Bioinformatics Company, taking its product to the top of Apple.com science downloads worldwide. He writes, and has appeared regularly, in major news-papers and a number of top business magazines, on the subjects of biotechnology, the environment and business strategy. He is the director of two companies and is currently co-founding a triple-bottom-line venture capital investment company. He is a sought-after speaker, mentor and facilitator on entrepreneurship, creativity and inspirational communication. Daniel has also been an actor for TV, film, and theatre. After a life-changing trip to India in 2006, where he found himself performing in a haka in front of 800,000 people, Daniel has dedicated his life to teaching the knowledge of a breathing technique to which he attributes every success in business, more importantly still, giving him an unshakable and stress-free happiness in the face of whatever life has thrown at him. www.bravishi.com www.bravishi.com/blogvishi

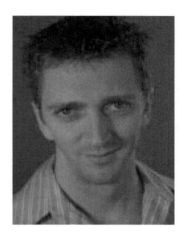

**Daniel:** Living my passion is actually about trust, faith and letting go of fear. It's waking up every single morning with a sense of excitement, knowing I'm doing something that I love, am good at, is aligned with my values, brings me joy to do, and gratitude to be in a position where I can do it. I want to provide models to others of different ways to do business, so I can be an example of someone who's doing business, not because I want to make screeds of money for myself, but to direct money skillfully into causes that matter in the world and the environment.

For a long time I had a belief I needed to do a whole lot of things that are not my passion first, in order to, maybe one day, get into a position where I can progressively get closer to something I'm passionate about doing. It took a while to realize this belief was a recipe for misery, because whatever you practice, you become! So if you practice doing things that are compromising, then you get good at being someone who compromises. If you become good at delaying the fulfillment of your true purpose in the world, then that's what you condition yourself to do. It's not as if one day you magically wake up after doing things you're not passionate about and you're suddenly in a position where you migrate to something you're passionate about. You will have had a whole history of living in fear in the meantime and you can't just suddenly turn that around.

## *The tipping point*

**Rose:** Do you ever come across any fear in yourself?

**Daniel:** Absolutely. It's always there. It's just a matter of not trying to deny it's there. If it's there, I just say: "Ok, there's fear here!" I know where it's coming from and remind myself that's not a true perception of the world. Normally the fear comes when I'm going back to a way of thinking which isn't Truth or Reality. I've come to understand this through spiritual learning. The more I'm in the spiritual world, the more I'm reminded, until I've basically reached a tipping point I suppose, where fear is still there, but it isn't the predominant way I look at the world. Fearful perception becomes the exception. Now, the principles of abundance, of synchronicity, serendipity, manifestation, these are the rhythms I live by on a day to day basis.

**Rose:** You notice the fear but you choose not to give it any weight?

**Daniel:** Yes, notice, don't judge, don't try to resist and it starts to move away. Then, as spiritual teachings show us, through the simple act of observation and not judging, you realize more and more, that's not a true reflection of how life is. For me that realization started when I read a book called *"The Artists Way"*, which to put it very simply, said: "Look we're all here to be creators. We're all creative." A basic principle of the Universe must be creativity. The Divine is exceptionally generous and abundant. There's not one flower created, but millions! The whole nature of the universe is incredibly rich and abundant with life, with beauty, with vitality, and it seems the wish of the Divine we find that abundance and creativity. It's just a simple, natural way of being. This is our nature.

**Rose:** To be divine?

**Daniel:** Exactly. We come into a false way of thinking, which is that the nature of the world is lack, and we need to struggle and put our own desires and joys on hold in order to do something sensible and right and all the rest of it. Sensible is part of it, but it's also meant to be sensational too!

What I'm passionate about is teaching the Art of Living, which is all about experiencing Oneness through something very tangible, which is the breath. Having done a lot of personal growth in the past, I've seen that can take you to the emotions, but there's a point beyond that we need to go to, on a level of trying to control this incredible thing called the mind, which wanders about all over the place, trips us up and says "oh, that's all very well but..", making excuses for our own actions. To control the mind, on the level of the mind, is impossible, but through the breath, you can actually control it. It's like the string on the end of a kite. As you pull the string, which is the breath, it uplifts the kite, and the same happens with the mind. It's a very powerful way we're all born with. It's here in our lungs. It's here in our body. The breath energises the body and through doing that, gives us a strong sense of ourselves. I encourage everyone to learn how to breathe, to learn how to meditate, and from these we get a sense of ourselves as we relate to other people. It helps us to be in community and to see some of the things that can otherwise get in the way of experiencing community: different egos, different personalities, different politics;

> ## Isabelle: A Caring Seed
>
> My WHOLE NEW WORLD seed would be a seed of caring. A world of Kindness, Love, Respect, Patience, Friendliness. Welcoming thoughts when greeted with a smile. Never lonely always friendly. Everyone will know what is good for him or her. Everybody will have a brighter future. A place where they belong. Almost like paradise. We will have freedom.

all tend to be less of an issue. A true perception of who we are allows us to be more truly in touch with other people and see them as they truly are. We don't have to react so much to something which may be pushing our buttons, but see it as some stress the other is expressing. Then we can see past our irritation, see who the other truly is and what's magical about them.

**Rose:** So for you, Oneness starts with the breath. What are you up to now, Daniel?

**Daniel**: One day a week I contract for a company I started three years ago with a friend, a hi-tech bio-information company which is now doing very well, selling to twenty markets internationally. I've recruited a new CEO, someone who can operate the business who is passionate about that sector, which is something I never was. Two days a week, I work on the "Art of Living" which is my absolute life purpose, to serve and give back the knowledge responsible for me gaining the peace of mind that enabled me to go into business in the first place. It has also given me the strength to go through some major traumatic life events and be strengthened by them rather than sunk by them.

As well, I'm also still serving through business, having developed skills in this area. I love the intellectual thrill, the principles of manifesting, being in a position where I can be a bridge between the business community and a spiritual way of living, acknowledging the spiritual world to the business community. I've learned the language of that community and I have a sense of how to communicate in terms understood by that community. I can act as a bridge for those people, who otherwise might not encounter such knowledge. This knowledge is not "mine" but comes through me from my spiritual teacher Sri Sri Ravi Shankar.

I'm in a position now, where more and more, business takes care of itself. Slowly and surely it's moving in that direction, so increasingly I have more time to give to activities which serve. The reason I do this is because I love it, because I'm passionate about it and it gives me great happiness to give back. I've realized what actually creates joy, is not the accumulation, but what you do with the resources and energy.

## *Ethics, environmentalism and enterprise*

**Rose:** When you serve, you experience joy, how wonderful! I under-stand you're planning to create a series of cds. Is your intention to help others to develop social entrepreneurship?

**Daniel:** I've heard social entrepreneurship used in many ways. It doesn't have to have a business component to it, whereas the cds are first and foremost a business proposition aimed at providing a company which is sustainable in three ways: commercially, environmentally, and to the community. It's a chance really to do several things. One is to create a product which is a stretch, something new to me and more creative. Two, it's the process of evolving the company which embodies the values of the product and three, it's looking at integrating what I call the three E's: **e**thics, **e**nvironmentalism and **e**nterprise, and really going beyond a dualistic way of looking at the world.

The Eastern mystical knowledge informs a lot of what I do. The dual-istic ways in which we look at the world, carve things up into black and white, right and wrong, manifest themselves in the ways we think without our realizing it. One of the dualisms we have is the left wing **o**r the right wing: I care about the environment and people **o**r I care about money. It's really as crude as that! What you have are different tribes or communities who attack each other's values rather than looking at points of commonality and seeing the oneness that under-lies all human experience. For me, there has to be a bigger container for the cultural and environmental, and that is the spiritual. It's not a mystical, go-and-chant-in-the Himalayas kind of thing. It's a very practical and pragmatic recognition of the Oneness of humanity. The knowledge does not come from me - I see my part simply as a bridge. I'm a vehicle for reminding people of what they already know, but have forgotten through a path we've been on since the Renaissance and possibly before, which is about carving up and dividing and specialising.

Two things in dualism, I'm looking to really meld together. On the one hand, we have a personal growth movement which is primarily apolit-ical, on the other hand, we have a political-environmental movement

which is focusing on the emotions of guilt and fear in order to motivate change. How can we combine something which is positive, love
driven, not fear driven and also has a very strong political, social and
greater good component to it, and see how they are not antagonistic
at all? They are deeply complementary. It's impossible to be realized
as a human being unless we're confronting the wider context of what
we're doing to the environment. It's impossible to be happy. That's
the starting point of the cd series: what does it mean to live in a way
which is empowered, empowering and acknowledging of some of the
problems in the world at the moment, in a way that doesn't go into
either denial or despair, but gives us a container of hope, joy, exhilaration and challenge?

**Rose:** That's what I call Love-in-action! How would a business structure
differ if you're working in a love-based model rather than a fear-based
model?

**Daniel:** Well, it's based on the principle of abundance. I think anyone
who's done extremely well in business always operates from this
principle: simply, that what you give comes back many times over.
You basically create your own reality. Whatever you think habitually
becomes your reality and thoughts will become a physical reality. I'm
looking at how nature sustains itself and modelling business based
on that. If you look at the human body, we take in air, which is 21%
oxygen, we breathe out 16% oxygen, so we're taking less than one
quarter of the oxygen from the air, and giving back the rest. If we
take slightly more than that, we wouldn't function so well. The body
is adapted to take in this optimal amount and it would be dangerous
and stressful to the body to take in more. If conversely, we take in less,
we very rapidly become tired and eventually will die, so there's an
optimal level of taking about 24% from the air and giving back 76%.
That's the model I'm using at the moment and experimenting with,
a business which is 76% focused on investigating intelligently how to
give back and 24% sustaining people who are in the business, so they
have enough oxygen, enough prana and life energy to sustain them;
so they're not getting exhausted. You can get into a poverty mentality
where you're giving everything and depleting yourself. There's a

delicate balance, and my intuition is it's about this level, because that's what nature does.

One of the things I love about business is that it's an environment in which to experiment and be quite honest and forthright about the areas you're experimenting with, but doing it in a context where you're not trying to reinvent the wheel. You're using those features of business which have worked extremely well in the past and are familiar, so you're not making it scary to people. It's still going to be a company. It's still going to have directors. It's still going to have reports, information, customers and a team, and all those good structural things. But anything which feels like fear will be eradicated. No person will have to do something they're not empowered to do, nor joyous about doing.

**Rose:** It's a social experiment really?

**Daniel:** It is, but I'm also looking at how it can still be something which is attractive to investors at the same time. Being very transparent to everyone about why it's being done, what the intentions are, where we see returns coming and why we think this will actually be much more profitable than anything coming from an old model; while also saying, "Look, business is not hard. Making profit is not hard. What's hard is doing it in a way that sustains people".

## Giving and receiving are one

Really, all I'm looking to do is to take business to another level and say: "How can we learn more about the process of giving, as we're building a new enterprise?" As opposed to just waiting until you've done nothing but accumulate. Remembering you become what you practice, why not actually practice the act of giving as you're building your enterprise and find novel ways that can be used, not only to get better at giving, but to create more abundance in the first place. I believe very much, the quality of what you create in your life is the quality of the questions you ask. If you ask questions like: "How can I possibly get a lot of money?" then it'll seem hard. But if you ask the question: "How can I possibly create a business which is so successful

I can afford to give away 75% and still be massively profitable?" then you're on the right track. You're asking the right question and the answer will be shown to you.

**Rose:** What you're saying is that our riches actually lie in community?

**Daniel:** It's nothing new. It's just going back to what we human beings are designed to do. That's live as social animals in a community and give to each other and, when we have more than we need, share it with the rest of the community. A year and a bit ago, I was quite resistant in some ways to the notion of community because of my negative associations with it from media images. Sometimes, these barriers and preconceived ideas stop us experiencing joy. It's the same with the word, spirituality. We have associations with that word, which don't actually reflect that truly spirituality is simply an experience of Oneness. I want to encourage people to go beyond the words, limitations and associations, and come back to a place of truth, which is really experiencing Oneness. Community and spirituality are the same because community is an expression of that Oneness with other people, that sense of belonging. The more we belong, the more our own power and responsibility increase.

# Leanne Holdsworth
## Optimistic about the human condition

Leanne Holdsworth is an independent consultant specialising in sustainable development and corporate social responsibility. She provides sustainability advice to a broad range of clients across the public and private sectors. She is the author of the book, *A New Generation of Business Leaders*, which studies Australian and New Zealand business leaders who have "done well by doing good". She is the mother of two small children and a board member for Enviroschools.

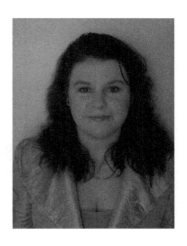

**Leanne**: When we talk about living our passion, for me, it's about influencing. The vehicle doesn't really matter too much. I tend to look for the place where there's most intersection between my skill and my passion. I think the drive underlying my passion is fairness and my response to injustice.

Living my passion is a continually evolving thing. I trained as a chartered accountant and worked in a chartered accounting firm for five years. In the end, I had to leave because what I valued was so different to the environment I was in and I felt so unsupported in the full expression of my authenticity at work. I was young, probably twenty four or maybe twenty five, when I experienced that, so rather than living my passion, I guess I ran away and lived in the country and thought, well, I'll have to explore something else. I don't know what my passion is, but it's definitely not this! It was while I was doing that for a few years, for the first time, I proactively found something I was passionate about. It was provoked by my attending a values-based leadership forum sponsored by Johnston and Johnston, for twenty eight to thirty two years olds. I had the opportunity of going there with another eighty young prospective leaders, and realized what I experienced in the chartered accounting scene was in fact a very familiar thing for young people to experience in the corporate world. There was harshness about the corporate world that didn't support our humanity. It was there I saw some work for me to do to change the work environment, which then prompted some years of work, and subsequently the book I wrote.

In my work creating work environments which are more humane for people's spirit, I added a dose of pragmatism after I'd written my book, and I ended up working for social responsibility in business.

It's been seven years since my book came out and there's been so much happening in that seven year period. The conversation about ethics and social responsibility in business arises so much more. The door is much more open today and I've been part of that change. I see endless possibility for the role of business, in terms of contributing to community and society, and to the future. Given the shift that's happened in the last seven years in business, there's a willingness to think more broadly than just making as much money as possible.

**Rose:** That must feel really good. I'm trying to feel into this a bit more in terms of how this change came about in the last seven years? Your book was possibly one of the catalysts, or it fed into something happening in the field? What else was influencing these changes?

**Leanne:** I suppose you could answer that in a number of ways. In one way it goes back to the '80's when there were several corporate catastrophes. Businesses lost money through being ignorant of what is important to stakeholders, be they their customers or civil society at large. Some multinationals found they were so out of step with civil society, their reputation and brand value were severely compromised. Business has learned some harsh lessons. When they ignore civil society, they won't fulfill their intention of making as much money.

Another influencing factor is, I think over time, people are more willing to have a voice. I'm completely optimistic about the human condition. Over time we become more incensed by injustice, but we also become more confused by detail and data. It's that tipping point, when a stage is reached, where things are clearly unfair, where human rights are being abused, when things have gotten so bad people will rebel and ask questions. Information is so much more readily available through the Internet. That's been a huge part of the shift of people being able to mobilise together quickly, globally, in reaction to something they don't want. The speed of being able to communicate globally affects how quickly people can decide to act, but there's just so very much more needing to be done!

**Rose:** There's an interesting polarity and tension between, on the one hand, you're working to heal injustice in the world, and on the other hand, you're feeling completely optimistic.

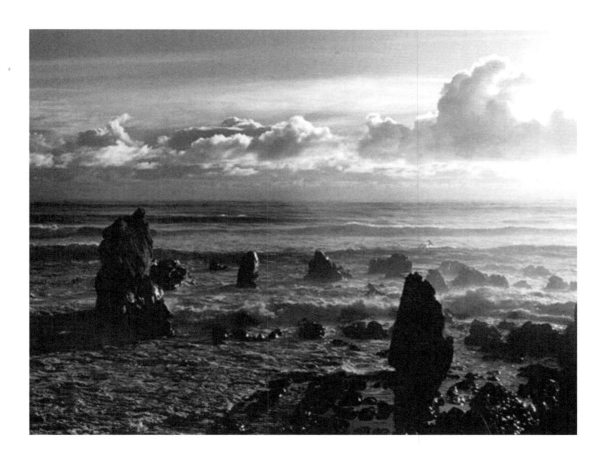

**Leanne:** I suppose when I look back, I think about the days of slavery and so on. We've become more intolerant. There are huge injustices even in our own country. Over time, we human beings are less willing to put up with these. In my own life I see so many things that need to be said or need to be done and I feel compelled to take responsibility for them. Living my passion is not a relaxing pursuit <u>and</u> I feel completely blessed to be able to support my family and do this at the same time.

**Rose:** One of the things that impresses me is you have managed to passionately pursue your cause of social justice within the mainstream and be successful there. Clearly, you've found a way to apply your passion and skills in a way that is acceptable.

**Leanne:** Thank you. I think as my passion changes, sometimes it becomes harder and harder to do this, because what I saw seven years ago was really the tip of the iceberg. I spend more time questioning, maybe business isn't completely the problem and we need to have a total overhaul of everything! If you think about an axis of, "institutionally everything's fine and we just tweak around the edges", at one end of the axis, and at the other end of the axis, "No, everything's completely wrong!" I've always been much more on the pragmatic end: let's make changes to what we've got. I think over time what's happened to me is I've become less tolerant of some of the tensions existing between, for instance, the role of business and social and environmental outcomes. I'm asking much more difficult questions which I suspect are going to end up making me less a friend of business and then things will be harder for me. I'm at the beginning of that really, not knowing how things are going to pan out. I think that's why I've become interested and involved in public policy.

**Rose:** I'm very impressed by what I've heard about the Caring Communities Project. What was the seed idea for this?

**Leanne:** When businesses are thinking about their social responsibilities, they often think about cause-related marketing or, in other words, what's going to add value to my business if I get involved with the community? In actual fact, the type of issues we have in the community, are not necessarily the ones a business might be attracted to. For instance, one of my particular areas of interest is domestic violence, and that's a very unattractive area for business. The Bank of New Zealand is now the sponsor of the organisation, Preventing Violence in the Home! This is fantastic, because it's not all about adding value to their brand.

The Caring Communities Project is not focused so much on what business does, as on all of us seeing where there are opportunities. Having been exposed to injustice through my work in domestic violence, I have an appreciation of things others can do to make it easier for victims and their families. When people don't know anything about domestic violence or child abuse because they're so far removed, it's very difficult for them to know what to do to help. It was important for me to introduce one section of the community to another as well as I could, to encourage everyone to participate, not simply let the businesses decide what areas were worthy of their investment.

**Rose:** It sounds like some of what you're doing is providing opportunities for deeper conversations to happen. The Caring Communities Project seems to open up possibilities in a relatively non-threatening way, and it's really up to the people where they take it. Do you have a sense things are really changing at the policy making level? Are policy makers seeing the social changes underway and responding to what is needed?

**Leanne:** No. I see huge opportunities for work to be done there.

**Rose:** Is it true to say the real transformation is occurring at the edges of society, but at the centre, there's no real awareness yet of the magnitude of changes needed?

**Leanne:** That's a difficult one. There are very, very smart people who've done lots of research around why we have poor social outcomes in some areas and there are some great little pilot projects happening, but there is such a lack of thinking, in a holistic sense, when policy is being designed. The ability for policy people to work together across functions, across professions, across ministries _and_ to be familiar with what life is like for most of the people involved, that level of understanding is so, so, so missing. With the Caring Communities Project, we're attempting to bring that level of understanding and yes, they know the statistics, and they know the facts, but they don't know what it's like! It's the bureaucratic problem of a well educated person trying to change the world without knowing what it's like to live in that world. You can't do that, I think, without a) working across disciplines bringing experts together and b) actually being there on the ground, in people's homes, having those conversations. That level of practical policy making doesn't happen very much yet.

**Rose:** Is that part of your current mission?

**Leanne:** Yep!

# *Shift Eleven*

## From concepts of "mine" and "yours", to recognition the Universe is a constant flow of energy, and giving and receiving are one.

Learning to work with universal flow is possibly one of the most invigorating aspects of the emerging culture and certainly one of the most challenging for Westerners, particularly when it comes to sharing money and resources. As social entrepreneurs lay the tracks for the emergence of a new culture based on universal principles and values, growing numbers of philanthropists are recognizing their part in supporting such projects, and together they are building new alliances which strengthen the web of community.

## EXTENDING COMMUNITY THROUGH CREATIVE RE-SOURCING AND PARTNERSHIP BUILDING

We cannot begin to consider a new culture without addressing the thorny question of money, a subject more divisive and less openly discussed than race, religion, or politics. Last year, some fifty or sixty co-creators were privileged to hear a talk by Catherine Austin Fitts, ex-Wall Street financier and ex Assistant Director of Housing for the United States government. She shared her understandings of how "the tape-worm system" of the global economy enables a few insiders to suck resources out of local communities leaving them vulnerable to crime and addiction. She advises people, who are worried about losing their fortunes on the stock market, to invest instead in local community ventures and businesses. This brings life and livelihood back into local communities and keeps wealth circulating for the common good. Different forms of community currencies have also been created and run successfully alongside the conventional monetary system.

Once the seed of a project has been planted, it needs watering with resources: money, a physical base, equipment, technological support, and so on. It is very difficult in New Zealand to find financial support in the early, creative stages of a project. For many transformational catalysts, Love-in-action involves faith, goodwill, a big generosity and a willingness to live simply. Working for years with little or no funding is not uncommon. Yet many of the people who are working this way are the hidden social architects of the future! Part of my hope for this book is that it will bring together social innovators with people who have the resources to help. My dream also is that this book will help to connect people and organisations from across the board, who will work together to make a difference. I would like to see "social entrepreneur" mean someone who can make a sustainable livelihood by creating social innovations and I would love to see these innovative ideas and practices move into the mainstream.

Robina spoke from the heart about how difficult it can be to find financial support:

**Robina:** The ground is generally not fertile in New Zealand, for my work. Maybe the conditions haven't become bad enough, or the visionary potential hasn't become strong enough, to receive what I create from my passion and back it with resources. I regularly end up being frustrated and feel like giving up in my own country. Whereas my experience in other countries like the USA or in Europe, where they see the writing on the wall, or in a country where there's more financial flow such as in Australia, or where there's desperate need, as in the Third World: at both extremes, my work is very well received, acclaimed and supported. Maybe it's that old idea that a prophet is never heard in her own land? Even though I have passion, even though I would love to give all the things I want to offer to this country, when I feel into the resonance, it's flat and dull and generally not singing in order to receive my gifts. I've been searching for probably twenty years already in my own country for that resonance frequency to resound. Generally I end up going it alone with very minimal resources, or using my own resources, working very creatively at the edge to bring heaps into being. It's like kneading my own dough, leavening my own bread. It comes from inside me; spirit and the fire of my passion move through me from my inner belly. Maybe this spirit of inspiration carries others along with me, because I'm definitely met by the right people at the right time, but there's some major ingredient missing. I get that ingredient when I work, for example in South Africa, where mountains move. There, everything is vital and electric! Here, there's a certain kind of sleepiness and dullness.

**Daniel** on the other hand, said:

If you look at what's happening in the USA, there is now a "Richest Fifty Philanthropists" list! Just imagine a script where you say: ok, the first and the second richest people in the world have given away over half their wealth to solving Third World diseases in Africa! You might say that's too unrealistic, but that's exactly what's happened and most wealthy billionaires in the US are now falling over themselves to find new, inventive ways of giving back. So it's very much in the zeitgeist right now. When people are asked why they're doing it they say: "I don't want to

*Dione:*
*A Kindness Seed*

*If I could I would plant the seed of Kindness. Kindness would change the world like no other, for example if people showed kindness to the environment there would be no global warming or pollution or toxic waste. Plus if people show kindness there would be no robberies because goods would be shared, and violence would be an ancient myth.*

ruin my kid's life." If you look at what happens when people inherit vast amounts of wealth, there's very good documented evidence that it ruins their life. So they're doing it for their children and they're doing it, because they want the joy of giving which they miss out on when they leave their estate to their lawyers to carve up after their death. They're realizing the true purpose of why they accumulate in the first place, which is to give their lives meaning and happiness. These three very compelling reasons have empowered a lot of people to be vastly philanthropic.

Just as there are people working at the grassroots, giving generously of their time and energy; there are also people willing to give generously of their financial wealth to support innovative projects. Is it simply a matter of making the links? This is a new and growing aspect of passionate service. You will find some New Zealand and global funding solutions and support for social entrepreneurs, in the Resources section at the end of the book.

# Culture Making

"We're beginning to become aware and it's a moment for actually giving birth to a new form of humanity. ....it is clear that we're called to do something monumental and magnificent."
—Brian Swimme, *The Universe is a Green Dragon*

*It's common to say that trees come from seeds. But how could a tiny seed create such a huge tree? Seeds do not contain the resources needed to grow a tree. These must come from the medium or environment within which the tree grows. But the seed does provide something that is crucial: a place where the whole of the tree starts to form. As resources such as water and nutrients are drawn in, the seed organizes the process that generates growth. In a sense the seed is a gateway through which the future possibility of the living tree emerges.*
—*Senge, Scharmer, Jaworski, Flowers,*
*Awakening Faith in an Alternative Future*

Passion is a fiery energy, and learning how to use the power of fire creatively has been a vital part of culture making since human life began. In psychological terms, the fire of passion exists on a continuum between destructive anger and the lust for power on the one end, and the refined and transmuted passion of service to a united world on the other.

We can easily see how these polarities are playing out on the world stage today. Humans have inhabited the planet for many thousands of years, yet as our creative powers increase, we are still very immature in our uses of fire. Maybe global warming, as well as being a fact we ignore at our peril, is a metaphor for what happens when collective consciousness swings too far to the angry pole, or when the container for our creative powers is not strong enough to hold and transmute our fire. The fire of nuclear explosion is another dark and potent metaphor of our times. Our human capacities for both creation and destruction are immensely powerful, yet so far, we have not developed sufficient collective love and wisdom to live in peaceful harmony with each other, with other living beings and with the Earth.

### Chelsea:
### A Kind Seed

*If I could sow a seed for a new world....the seed would be a kind seed where everyone helped one and other. People would not have problems with people from other cultures just because they were from a different country and if people were a different religion from their friends, they would respect their friend's religion too.*

The passion of anger and greed is expressed through the dynamic of power-over, domination, and control. I believe this is what people mean when they speak of "the old energy". This egocentric, driven, pushing, grabbing energy cannot tolerate difference, becomes violent when thwarted, and will ruthlessly destroy anything which stands in its way. Anyone who has ever been very angry will be able to find this energy in themselves. It is ugly and therefore unpleasant to identify with and own. We'd prefer to believe all the ugly stuff belongs to the bad guys over there, the ones who are different from us, the ones who are destroying the world.

Could this be the time for a collective new beginning? Perhaps a little collective humility is timely in the face of the mystery of our creative powers and our infinitesimal place in the cosmos.

What if the world can only be healed within each one of us? What if our willingness to journey deep into the self and deep into our relationships, to heal the self, creates a new space in which a whole new world can come into being through us?

On the opposite pole from power-over, we find power-with, or the dynamics of partnership and co-creation. This is a dynamic of attraction, curiosity and inventiveness. When we live our passion, we follow what is attractive to us and are curious to enter the unknown, to explore, discover, and invent the new. When we are attracted by love, creativity and expanded consciousness, we give ourselves to the fire of transformation. Consciously choosing to co-create with the evolutionary power of universal intelligence, we surrender our lower vibration energy to be refined by the flames. We bring our unique gifts, life experience and resources into play with the universal originating force, to create something at once totally new, and yet at the same time, building on everything which has gone before. When we co-create with another, or with a group of others, we each bring our own special part, our own unique perspective, and find in the doing, how these parts fit together, where the resonance is, how together we can discover and invent.

The interviews in this book point towards a new emerging culture built on the foundation of shared values. For Jonathan, these values are expressed in the choice between life giving or life taking actions. For Donna, the choice is between love and fear. Underlying all action is respect for the sacredness of all Life and being in service to our interconnection with all that lives.

As I think about building a new culture, I am imagining a house without walls, built for an ever expanding community. The **foundation stone** is our relationship with nature, with the awesomely abundant, generous, diverse creativity of our beautiful planetary home; with the earth, air, water and fire, from which we are formed and which sustain us. This gives rise to global responsibility and the shared values of:

*LIVING IN SERVICE TO HUMANITY,*
*PLANET EARTH AND ALL LIVING SYSTEMS*

*HONOURING THE INTERCONNECTEDNESS*
*AND SACREDNESS OF ALL LIFE*

*EVOLVING THROUGH EXPERIENTIAL LEARNING*

To build the **container** for our new culture, I envisage **four pillars**:

*INNER WORK*

*CONSCIOUS RELATIONSHIP*

*LIVING OUR PASSION AS LOVE-IN-ACTION*

*CO-CREATIVE COMMUNITY*

For the roof of our new global meeting place, I envision our relationship with the mystery of cosmos, which is within and beyond us. This includes:

*A SHARED STORY OF OUR ORIGINS AND THE EVOLUTION*
*OF THE NEW UNIVERSAL HUMAN*

*A CREATION-CENTRED SPIRITUALITY*

A full exploration of this framework for a new culture is beyond the scope of this book. However, such a framework could create a container within which the alchemy of personal, social and global transformation can manifest. I would love to see this framework at the centre of every curriculum, in every educational establishment, from pre-school through to universities. Imagine the kind of world we would live in if this were the case!

There's a new, authentic, universal human, consciously co-creating with evolutionary universal intelligence and coming together with others in new collective forms. This book and all the people in it, point towards a Whole New World based on the understanding that all life is one interconnected whole.

The world's young people are our greatest hope. I am deeply inspired by the conscious contributions of David and Kat, both in their twenties.

There are many other young people I would have loved to include, who are equally brilliant. The children also have wise and creative things to say about the future they want to create. But how much of a world will be left for them, if society at large, does not change now, and who is responsible to make sure positive change happens?

This last section explores three important aspects of a new culture:

**Chris and Takawai Murphy** talk about Pumaoamo, the course they have developed, which advocates a partnership model to raise awareness and improve race relations between Maori and Pakeha (European) New Zealanders. They remind us how important it is to preserve the diversity of the world's cultures. The knowledge, wisdom and identity held in Maori language, songs and protocol, come from the land, are of the land, and contribute to personal and national identity and self-esteem. Modelling partnership beautifully themselves, Chris and Takawai's message to respect and honour differences would support any partnership. A move toward co-creative global community based on the principle of unity in diversity, starts with the healthy self-esteem and self expression of individuals, and preserves the essence of all the different cultures with which our world has been blessed.

**Jim Horton and Susan Jessie:** Meaningful rituals to honour life transitions have been mainly lost from Western culture. Jim and Suzi share how their rites of passage programmes: Tracks, for young men and Tides, for young women, have evolved from the practice of living together in intentional community, from being parents, and from their passion for growing strong, distinctive men's and women's gatherings. In this interview, they extend a heartfelt challenge to us to value our young people. Their ground-breaking work demonstrates how self-esteem, personal and group empowerment, inter-generational understanding and communication, can be built and sustained in ways that provide gifts of the heart to all involved and contribute to a culture of nonviolence.

**Vivienne Anne Wright** is deeply committed to One People One Planet; a New Zealand based global initiative for creating a peaceful, sustainable world by connecting children into a pro-active global community of Peace Pals. Working for nearly five years without funding, Vivienne has succeeded in bringing together the support of experts drawn from many different disciplines and fields, both within New Zealand and overseas. Children are already actively involved in a number of creative projects and very enthusiastic about the opportunity to become agents of peace. As Vivienne says, the future belongs to the children. This remarkable and empowering initiative is scattering seeds of hope and promise to the winds of the future. It is truly an example of dedicated, globally responsible leadership and creative alliance-building.

# Living your passion means:

*I see language as a taonga (treasure) providing me with access to the stories and traditions, the wisdom of my people. It has meant reclaiming the karakia (incantations, conversations with the Gods) of our ancestors, learning the spiritual songs. Along the journey, I have grown and continue to grow in my appreciation and identification with my Maori cultural heritage. I have a desire to help others see the values and beliefs embedded within this cultural context. —Takawai*

*We can bring people together rather than divide them. We need to be more united for the very survival of our planet. We should all be looking for ways to improve our relationships with Earth and all people. —Chris*

*The truth is, when you take that boy through a process where he now becomes a young man, and he's valued and recognized by his community and honoured, and you invite him back to the event as a young leader, what we call a tracker, to help the next lot of new boys to come through; in other words, you put him into a servant leadership role, he is so there with his heart! They come from their hearts! It's brilliant! It's amazing how much they want to help! —Jim*

*Maybe my passion is being a midwife, not in the conventional sense, but more in the sense of raising seedlings, whether they're kids or plants or whatever, and helping them to grow to their full potential. —Suzi*

*Right now I am in a place where my elemental desire is to know I'm making a difference at a time when the planet is at a pivotal stage in its evolution. I look into the future with a great deal of optimism. I believe we can achieve much if we come together on a commonly agreed platform of respect and sharing and work together towards a commonly agreed goal. It is time to find new ways of living together in harmony, with the greater good of all, our major objective. —Vivienne*

# *Shift Twelve*

## The realization of Unity

We come to understand at a conceptual and intuitive level that every living being is connected into one indivisible and interdependent web of Life. Over time, and with meditative practice, this becomes an experiential, moment to moment realization of the Unity of all life. Or, a sudden peak experience may reveal this unity, and then we strive to integrate this new understanding with our established world view.

# Chris and Takawai Murphy
## When the Bellbird and the Tui sing together

Chris and Takawai met as student teachers in 1969 and married in 1971. They live in Ngaruawahia, North Island, New Zealand. They have two children, Enoka and Ngahuia and five grandchildren. They have both worked in education for the whole of their adult lives, and have both held senior positions in schools. They continue to work together, facilitating Nationhood Building seminars throughout Aotearoa - New Zealand. takawai@xtra.co.nz

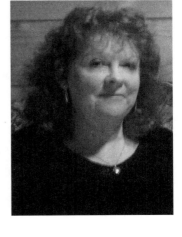

A couple of years ago, I participated in a wonderful workshop, called *Te Pumaomao: A Nationhood Building Strategies and Solutions Course*. At the time, I was doing research into New Zealand history and Maori mythology for the second edition of my first book, Migration to the Heartland, and I went along hoping to learn something about the early migrations. The two day course was held at the local marae, or Maori meeting house, where we all spent the night sleeping "marae style", side by side in one big room, decorated with Maori art, breathing the same breath. The course turned out to be exceptionally good. It was led by Chris and Takawai Murphy, wife and husband, she Pakeha and he Maori. The focus of their work is on promoting partnership between the two

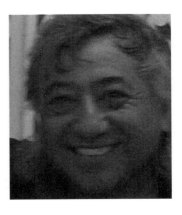

races. Years before, I had attended a "Te Tiriti o Waitangi" workshop, obligatory for anyone teaching in New Zealand. Te Pumaomao included the Treaty and it was participatory, fun, informative, nonthreatening and deeply moving. For me, it was a transformational experience; by the end of our two days together, I had had an experience of Unity.

**Takawai:** Apart from my family, the work I do through *Te Pumaomao* is the most important thing in the world to me. To be able to live it every day, as a job, although it can be tiring and energy draining, is absolutely brilliant.

**Chris**: For Takawai, Te Pumaomao is part of him; it's his story, his history. The importance of expressing that history to others in a way that perpetuates understanding and good will is vital. Takawai also has a real passion for trying to help his people reclaim their identity and be proud of who they are. I enjoy the work as well. It gives our life meaning and a sense of purpose.

**Rose:** That sounds very total, as if nothing of you is left out, Takawai. I believe the programme is something you've created yourself? Can you tell me a bit about how it came about and how it has evolved?

**Takawai**: It came about in the 1980's, when I was a school teacher and I could see Maori kids didn't get the same opportunities to succeed in schools as other kids. Pakeha kids had the right to receive an education, justice, health and so on, in their mother tongue, in a system created by them, run by them, under their norms, mores, and protocols. I thought Maori, if they were equal, should be entitled to the same, with an education in their language and designed by them. As a teacher, if you thought like that back in those days, you were classified as a radical and an activist, and life became very uncomfortable. So I decided it would be better for me to get out of school teaching and work out a way to help others see where Maori people like me were coming from.

I spent five years of my spare time putting together a teaching programme to achieve my aim. I had a lot of help from both Maori and Pakeha people. One was a Pakeha nun, Sister Genevieve, who was inspirational as well as being a huge support. Once I got the programme prepared, I started teaching it full time. That was in 1990.

I was fortunate that the Nursing Council was getting into teaching cultural safety to student nurses and there wasn't a lot of knowledge in that area, so I got my first job at the Polytechnic, teaching cultural safety to nurses. There was also a need for other Polytechnic students to have some Treaty knowledge. I was lucky, when I went to work in this area, I had a ready market. And it grew from there.

**Rose:** I found your programme very heartfelt.

**Chris**: It *is* heartfelt because it's real. It deals with a perspective that has often been overlooked or misunderstood.

**Rose**: I'm sure there will be people outside New Zealand reading this book, could you say briefly why the Treaty of Waitangi is so important to New Zealanders and Maori in particular, at this time?

**Takawai**: The Treaty is extremely important in that it provides a framework for the future. It details what the political, social, environmental, and economic relationship should look like between Maori and Pakeha: equal status and authority. At the time the treaty was signed, in 1840, Maori outnumbered Pakeha by one hundred to one, and the Maori attitude was: "Although our numbers are large and yours are small, we have equal status, equal authority, and equal mana"; in other words, "partnership". Maori have a whakatauki (proverb) about it, which says:

*"Ko koe ki tena, ko au ki tenei kiwai o te kete"*
*"You take that handle of the basket,*
*I'll take this one, and we'll share the load together."*

Maori still think like this today, even though the numbers have been reversed and Pakeha now outnumber Maori.

The Treaty also spells out clearly that Maori would retain total authority over the land and other resources. It was designed by humanitarians, so that what had happened to other indigenous peoples would not happen to Maori. Even though the Treaty has never been honoured by their treaty partner, it still provides a positive blueprint for the future, for Maori and justice-driven non Maori to strive to achieve.

**Rose:** You've given a very clear and helpful summary of what I know to be contentious issues. Are you mainly running your workshop with Pakeha, or with Maori also? And do you notice any difference when you're running it for one or the other group?

**Takawai:** We run our course for any group who request it and, as it works out, about one third of the courses are for Pakeha groups, one third are for Maori groups and one third are for mixed groups. There's also a course we run each year for migrants and one for Boston University (USA) students as well. We have a lot of immigrants attend through courses we facilitate for staff of City Councils, District Health Boards, and other organisations.

**Chris:** For a Maori group, it is different. They know the stories. They are their stories, and we're putting them into a framework they can easily relate to. For Pakeha groups, it's neat too, because, for the majority, there are new understandings from a perspective they haven't heard before. A lot of issues they have been confused about, start falling into place. Migrants are great too, because they're open to learning. We always try hard to keep every person safe within the challenge of new learning.

**Rose:** It sounds like the main purpose behind Te Pumaomao is personal and cultural empowerment?

**Chris:** Yes. It's about enlightenment through creating a new understanding. Hopefully, some of those long held fears and anxieties about race relations will dissipate. It's multidimensional, really.

**Takawai:** Yes. It's about empowering Maori to be able to make more informed decisions about learning the language, reclaiming treasures which were nearly lost, and being able to stand proud as Maori. Many, aged forty plus, have grown up in a society which conditioned them to believe everything Maori was second rate and inferior to Pakeha. Our course is about correcting that kind of conditioning.

For other New Zealanders, it's about empowerment to be able to understand the situation. In their upbringing, they were fed countless myths about Maori. Our course gives them information to counter the myths and teaches them history from a Maori perspective, so they are able to understand what the issues are. It enables them to look beneath the surface, when issues arise in the media. We're not saying there is only one perspective; participants take from the course what they are comfortable with. It also empowers them with the knowledge to question. For example, they start to examine social indicators and begin to see maybe they reflect something not so healthy in our society, rather than just blaming Maori for figuring so disproportionately in negative statistics.

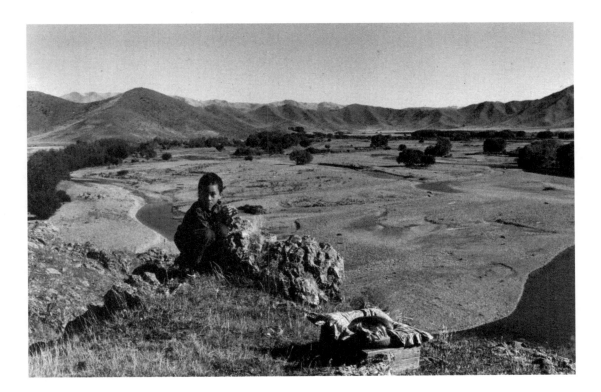

**Chris**: In other words, they get to form a critical perspective.

**Rose:** Takawai, I remember you talking about how this has been a personal journey for you in terms of your own empowerment and understanding?

**Takawai:** Yes, over quite a long period of time, I reclaimed a lot of things for myself and that's been an enlightening process; fulfilling and rewarding.

*"Tirohia kia marama, whawhangia kia rangona te ha!"*
*Observe to gain enlightenment, participate to feel the essence.*

I started out not being able to speak the language. Now I can do that! I see language as a taonga (treasure) providing me with access to the stories and traditions, the wisdom of my people. It has meant reclaiming the karakia (incantations, conversations with the Gods) of our ancestors, learning the spiritual songs. Along the journey, I have grown and continue to grow in my appreciation and identification with my Maori cultural heritage. It has also impacted me in the way I think about the land, the sea and the natural environment. I have a desire to help others see the values and beliefs embedded within this cultural context. It's been a huge journey! We're lucky our two kids have been a part of it as well. They're now adults and into the same kinds of things as we are.

**Rose**: I'm hearing that learning the Maori language was an important part of your process. Can you tell me what it's like to walk in both worlds?

**Takawai:** Being able to speak my mother tongue is wonderful. My sense of being Maori is enhanced. I'm now able to participate in conversations and fulfill any protocol task confidently. Language is an integral part of who we are. I also feel the responsibility for doing my part to help keep the language alive.

Having a greater understanding, knowledge, and ability in te reo (Maori language), has helped me feel complete as a person. I feel secure from within and this also allows me to participate confidently in both worlds.

**Rose**: An important aspect of your course is your emphasis on partnership. Working together, you beautifully model partnership between Maori and Pakeha, a man and a woman. You're really walking the talk! I know co-working isn't always easy and you do it very well, working side by side to create something better than either could do alone.

**Takawai:** Yes. The biggest decision I made was about eight years ago when I asked Chris to work with me. At the time, I was working away from home, she was staying at home and we had no kids at home. I suggested we work together as a team and it's been absolutely brilliant! Two heads are better than one and she can sit back and evaluate. Since she's worked alongside me, we've made immense changes to the programme and improved it heaps. We're lucky we're best mates, so we never ever have any strife working together.

**Chris:** We're easygoing in many ways. Now and then, I'll fire up, but it doesn't happen very often. I think it's good for others to see how easy it is, and for me to be able to give another viewpoint from Takawai's. But even within our different views, there is respect and understanding and I think people can see that.

**Rose:** What would you say is the essence of good race relations?

**Chris:** Flexibility, understanding, open-mindedness, respect, and the ability to realize we can get along. Some people think it's difficult, but I know that it's not. It is the human factor we all have in common. Our humanness brings us together. It's not so bad to have different perspectives. We don't all have to be the same. We don't have to agree on every single issue. That's not natural. There's no threat in seeing things differently. To me it's easy. I respect who Takawai is, I understand his journey and have no worries about it. There are a lot of other things too that come into it: knowledge, appreciation of another person's history, balancing, and heaps of subtleties. On the surface, that is what it means to me. You first have to understand the history and accept other people have had different histories, different values and belief systems from your own and that it is okay. Once you can accept this, then you begin to move on in positive directions.

**Rose:** These qualities sound like a foundation for any good partnership. Perhaps good race relations are simply an extension of good partnership? Yet it seems to be part of human nature to be afraid of difference.

**Chris:** I think it's a psychological legacy from eons back when perhaps difference was a threat, and as we evolve, maybe the fear will dissipate altogether. The younger generations are a wee bit more flexible than we were.

**Takawai:** It's important to accept there's not only one way of doing things. It's all about acceptance that to speak another language is ok. It's about accepting we can be good friends and get on really, really well as Maori and Pakeha, as long as there is respect for Maori speaking their own language and doing things their own way.

**Chris:** It's also an appreciation that things done differently have their own wisdom. Maori have karakia (incantations, conversations with the Gods) for certain seasons of the year. They have their proverbs (whakatauki), little encapsulated bits of wisdom from the ancestors, which are still appropriate today. You know, there is a lot of knowledge that is really amazing and different.

**Rose**: It's really important to keep that alive, isn't it?

**Chris:** Yes and the course is about keeping that knowledge alive and encouraging others to do so.

**Rose:** I came to New Zealand about twelve years ago from the UK, so I'm a relative newcomer. For me, there's something incredibly powerful about the land itself. There seems to be a deep spiritual essence in the land. I imagine much of Maori knowledge and wisdom pertains to the power of the land?

**Takawai:** Maori have a strong affinity with the land. The land is Papatuanuku, the Earth Mother, who nurtures and sustains us. There's a real intertwining between nature and people. For example, the people from Whanganui have a saying:

*"Ko au te awa, ko te awa ko au"*
*"I am the river, the river is me".*

When a baby is born, Maori return the placenta, the afterbirth (the whenua), to the land (the whenua). To Maori, the placenta and the land are both considered whenua, that's how strong the connection is!

**Rose:** That connection is so essential! The materialistic Western culture has tried to make everything the same. It's tried to get rid of all the differences, to colonise and destroy all the different cultures, even to the extent of extinguishing so many species of wildlife and animals; so much of the beautiful diversity of the planet. It seems so crucial for the future of everyone that the differences and wisdom of indigenous cultures are preserved.

**Takawai:** Yes for sure, and wrapped up within those indigenous languages and cultures are some really good answers about caring for the environment and for people doing things in better ways. Globalisation is making everyone and everything the same. It's killing these different kinds of knowledge.

**Rose:** I imagine there's a delicate balance between wanting to share that knowledge and yet wanting to preserve it. How do you keep something sacred and share it at the same time?

**Takawai:** I think for those non Maori who look to live the life, they get access to the treasures, to information and knowledge, simply because they're there in a supportive way and they're accepted and trusted by Maori. It's amazing how much sacred knowledge our old people share with my wife, Chris, because they accept her, trust her and know she's an ally. But because the majority of non Maori don't walk in that world, they often don't understand there are treasures.

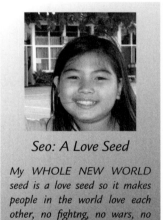

*Seo: A Love Seed*

My WHOLE NEW WORLD seed is a love seed so it makes people in the world love each other, no fightng, no wars, no killing.

**Rose:** I believe a central idea of Maori culture is that Maori are guardians of the land, or kaitiaki. Could you say something about that?

**Takawai:** Yes, the Treaty of Waitangi recognized Maori were the kaitiaki (guardians) of the land and promised them they would retain that status for as long as they wished. Our role as kaitiaki is to preserve the land and care for it for "nga uri whakatipu" (for the next generation), and their role is to do the same. Unfortunately, our Treaty partner began passing laws to take that status from Maori and to transfer it to themselves.

**Rose:** It seems there are many seeds of a new culture growing and being planted at the moment in Aotearoa. I'm wondering what your vision is for the future, from the perspective of the work you do.

**Chris:** It's mainly about hope and acceptance of difference, preserving aspects of the Maori culture and keeping it sacred.

**Takawai:** To me the vision is that both peoples (Maori and non Maori) are able to achieve their dreams and their aspirations in their own way. They're not forced into each other's systems, if they don't work for them. For example, Maori won't be forced into a Pakeha education system if we know that clearly doesn't work for us. (50% of Maori boys leave school with no qualifications). It will be a society where there are choices and options.

**Chris**: It is also about making systems more proactive and supportive, so that non Maori adjust as well.

**Rose**: Having different systems working alongside each other whilst accepting and respecting the differences?

**Chris:** Differences within systems too. Maybe it's about being willing to look at doing things in new ways, rather than repeating the old stuff that isn't working. Testing and evolving, rather than accepting the status quo. That's bigger than us, but for us, it's about sowing the seeds of positive transformation.

**Rose:** Earlier you were talking about identity and I guess a strong sense of identity is central to all of this? It's easier to accept differences when we have a strong sense of who we are. Then we feel less threatened by someone's different identity.

**Chris:** I think that's exactly right.

**Takawai:** Many non Maori New Zealanders are not strong in their own cultural identity. When they're not strong, they may feel challenged and threatened by Maori. I think part of the growing process is for non Maori to learn about themselves.

This can be achieved by making Aotearoa – New Zealand history a core component of the curriculum in education. Until non Maori become strong in their own identity, it's going to make it difficult to progress in accepting Maori, who are strong in theirs..

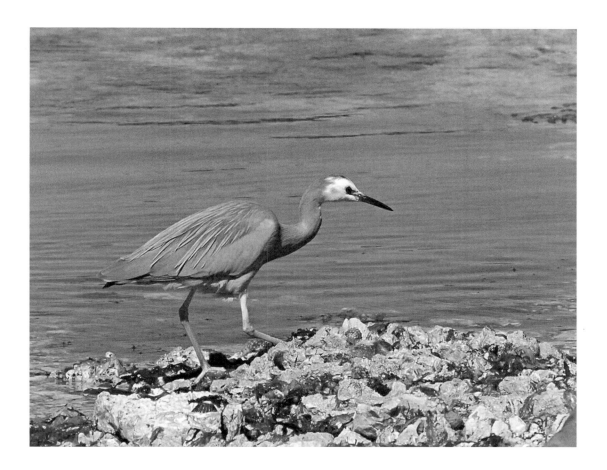

# *I AM MAORI*

*Am I Maori?*
*Yes I am,*
*for I have brown skin.*
*Am I Maori?*
*Yes I am, they say,*
*for I have curly, black hair.*
*Am I Maori?*
*No, my language has been replaced.*
*Am I Maori?*
*No, my language is English.*
*Am I Maori?*
*Yes I am,*
*for now is the awakening,*
*stirring deep inside my soul,*
*arising, arising, arising,*
*seeping through this Pakeha mist*
*of many years,*
*penetrating the concrete walls,*
*reaching down to the rich brown earth*
*encased underneath.*
*Stirring, stretching, reaching*
*reaching for that tiny seed*
*of Maoridom in an ancient past.*
*No, not all is lost.*
*I am becoming Maori.*
*I will not lose what I am,*
*what I am awakening to.*
*Am I Maori?*
*Yes, my heart is telling me so,*
*crying:*
*I am Maori.*

*Hinewirangi Kohu: Broken Chant Poems,*
Rosemary Kohu and Robert de Roo, The Tauranga Moana Press 1983, 1984

**Rose:** Many of us in the West have lost a strong connection to our cultural roots, and growing numbers look to indigenous cultures, like Maori or Native Americans, for example, to teach us about ritual, connection with nature, natural medicine, or our place in the cosmos.

**Takawai:** To Maori, cultural roots are everything, so you learn your whakapapa (genealogy), and your identity markers:

*Ko Tawhiuau te maunga.* Tawhiuau is the (my) mountain.

*Ko Rangitaiki te awa.* Rangitaiki is the (my) river.

*Ko Ngati Manawa te iwi.* My people are Ngati Manawa.

*Ko Apa Tangiharuru te tupuna.* Apa Tangiharuru is the founding ancestor of my people.

Every iwi (tribe) has its own whakatauki (proverbs), karakia (incantations) and waiata (songs) which are unique to them and which celebrate their cultural roots. One of those whakatauaki (proverbs) is occasionally recited to those living in the cities, away from their tribal homelands:

> *Hoki koe ki to maunga kia purea ai koe e nga hau o Tawhirimatea"*
> *Return to your mountain to be cleansed by the winds of Tawhirimatea,*
> *(god of the winds).*

As Maori reclaim those treasures, almost lost through colonisation, they are also returning to 'rongoa', those medicines concocted from the native trees and plants around them.

Once again, they are celebrating the Cosmos. Every year now Matariki, the Maori New Year is celebrated (in June). Matariki is a constellation of stars known to the English as The Seven Sisters, to the Japanese as Subaru and astronomically as Pleiades!

**Chris:** I think many of us, although not strong in our cultural identity, still have some affinity with our past, our roots. However, I do think the knowledge other cultures offer is becoming more accepted and appreciated, and perhaps sought after by some.

**Rose:** One of the things I remember from your workshop was the theme of colonisation, and of course, part of the legacy of New Zealand history is the colonisation of Maori culture by Pakeha, just as this happened in many other parts of the world with other cultures. I'm a white Westerner, so on the one hand, I come from the people who have been colonisers, on the other hand, my English ancestors were rural peasants and artisans and then slaves of the industrial revolution. If you go further back, there was the destruction of the Goddess religion, which was a religion of the Earth, of the soul, and of the interconnection of Life. Colonisation is still going on under the tyranny of multinational globalisation and the kind of monoculture that's been imposed on us. I know and understand both sides: what it is to be colonised and what it is to be part of an oppressive culture.

**Chris:** I think it's important to come to an acceptance too, of things that have happened in history, that haven't been quite right. I don't carry any guilt over this. It's important to lose the guilt and think positively about how we can make a difference. The lessons are always there to be learnt from our history, but we often repeat the self-defeating cycles.

**Rose:** So, it's about letting go of the hurts and betrayals of the past and moving forward with love and forgiveness?

**Chris:** Yes, moving forward in new ways, different from the past.

**Takawai:** I think it's about fixing things up in a way that's fair and just, and moving forward in positive ways, where we don't repeat the wrongs of the past. Unfortunately, we're not quite getting that right. Just this week the United Nations issued a report containing twenty two concerns and recommendations. It continues to criticise the Foreshore and Seabed Act and strongly urges the Government to enhance the status and recognition of the Treaty.

It's about not feeling guilty for the things that have been done in the past, but fixing them up in a just way. I think it's going to be pretty hard to do, although we have started the process. If you look at the parallel education system Maori have started, it shows we're firmly on the journey. I think the Treaty settlements are a start as well. The journey has begun, but it will take a while to complete.

**Rose:** What you've said is such clear wisdom for us all: to come to terms with the past, to be present and respectful, and to move forward into the future in a new way. This is real, clear, simple wisdom; yet so hard to do! *Laughter.*

**Takawai:** Yes, easy to say and difficult to achieve! I think it is possible though and it's starting to happen! I've noticed young Pakeha people coming out of university are much more open and accepting of difference than their predecessors. Change is underway but it will take time.

**Rose:** I had a very strong feeling of Oneness or Unity after your course. I truly had the experience we are all actually One. So how can we preserve difference whilst experiencing Oneness! With the way the planet is at the moment, this seems vitally important, if we're to evolve.

**Takawai:** Yes, we have a beautiful land here in New Zealand. People want to come and live here. We've clearly got something really, really good. I'd like to see us building a healthier society that is more accepting of difference and offering many choices and options. Underneath that, there's recognition everyone is the same. I reckon that's the secret.

**Rose:** Could you remind me of what Te Pumaomao means?

**Takawai:** It means: "Reflecting on the Past, Making Provision for the Future." It's a Nationhood Building Strategies and Solutions Course.

**Rose:** That's a wonderful idea, building nationhood, then perhaps going beyond nation to recognize we are One World?

**Chris:** I guess that's part of the vision too; we can bring people together rather than divide them. We need to be more united for the very survival of our planet. We should all be looking for ways to improve our relationships with Earth and all people.

**Takawai:** When you look at all the problems in the world today, clearly there's a need for this kind of course to help nations resolve their issues in nonviolent ways.

**Rose:** New Zealand is such a multicultural nation now, isn't it?

**Chris:** Yes, yet it's important to preserve the essence of the country. If we went to France, it still has the essence of France, which is different from the essence of Italy or Germany. If we went to Japan, there's still an essence of Japan. Even though New Zealand may be more multicultural, this is a recent thing. There is something much deeper, a history that has its own meaning and relevance. It's about preserving that, not about rejecting multiculturalism and the benefits it brings.

**Rose:** What lies beneath the New Zealand culture is the unique essence of the land; an indigenous culture is harmonious with the land.

Thank you again for your course. Talking with you now, I'm remembering all its different layers: the Treaty of Waitangi, the suffering of colonisation, the history of New Zealand, and the hope of genuine partnership. I found it a very profound transformational experience; it opened up in me the inner knowledge that we are all One People, even though we are all different and have our different ways.

**Chris:** I remember standing outside the marae in Golden Bay listening to Takawai's whaikorero (speech) and hearing the bellbird and the tui sing at the same time. That is magical! You don't often hear them together. It is all about allowing us to sing together in different ways; appreciating different identities; recognizing the past still has a presence in today; understanding that the effects of the past are still needing to be healed; and moving on in positive ways.

**Rose:** It was very special too, doing the course at the marae. Each time I've been on a marae, it's been a very special experience, creating a greater sense of Oneness. Marae have such heart energy.

**Takawai:** History too. Maori say: *"You're not standing alone, you're standing with many. The room is full."*

# *PAST/FUTURE*

*Yesterday*

*Stands clearly in sight*

*My ears*

*hear many calls*

*You cannot live in the past*

*Conclusions of another race*

*-the Pakeha past is behind*

*but the Maori*

*past lies beside the future and is now!*

*Our past*

*builds mana*

*Takitimu builds strength*

*In the Maori world*

*ancestors teach*

*me to grow*

*whakapapa*

*dignity*

*pride*

*spiritual travel*

*customs*

*values*

*gods/goddesses teach*

*love of life*

*land*

*sea*

*air*

*- that is my mauri,*

*creating me,*

*moulding me,*

*pulling from my very depth*

*the Maori spirit.*

*Screaming Moko* by Hinewirangi Kohu: the Tauranga Moana Press 1986

# Jim Horton and Susan Jessie
## You are a seed! You're germinating!
## You're flowering! You're unfolding!

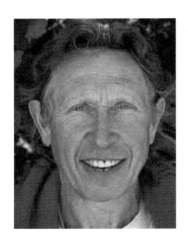

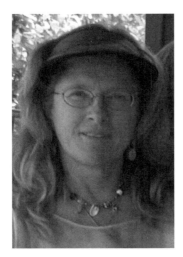

**JIM HORTON**: I am from England and have lived in South Africa and Canada, where two of my sons were born. After living in New Zealand for fifteen years I now consider it my home. I was a dentist for thirty years. Now in my early sixties, I have spent the last thirteen years actively involved in the men's culture which I have played a part in growing here, as well as in Australia, South Africa, Canada, and the USA. I am the father and step-father of five grown boys and this, and the fact I have lived in intentional community with several other families of kids growing up around me, is one of the main triggers that initiated TRACKS. My personal journey with men's work led me to the concept of Conscious Mentoring and "Rites of Passage" (Initiation) over eight years ago. Since then, I have also become interested in the concept of "Eldership" in our modern society, fostering a generational men's culture that supports the growth of healthy people. I am an active Trustee of the Tui Spiritual and Educational Trust and I live in Tui Community, Golden Bay, with my partner Susan Jessie, our dog Maggie, and several small fish. suzijim@tracks.net.nz

**SUSAN JESSIE**: I live in New Zealand, though I was born in Leeds, England, where my father was doing extra medical study. With my parents and older sister, I returned to New Zealand when I was three and settled in Wellington, where

I spent my teenage years. I am now moving into the second half of my life, a wonderful place to be and a time to return the gifts, nourish my creativity and deepen into my own silences. I am the mother of three sons and the stepmother of two more. I have been living at Tui Community now for fifteen years, and over this time have witnessed the unfolding into adulthood of my own and other children here. Through this experience, I came to recognize the need to mark times of transition consciously, and the importance of rites of passage, starting at birth and finishing at death, with other major transitions in between. In the world where I grew up, these transitions were not acknowledged and instead we created our own, often around the misuse of drugs and alcohol. When someone suggested starting a programme for young women, called Tides, for girls transitioning into young women, I decided it was important to be on board. I am now the co-ordinator of this programme. This was a natural step from co-facilitating women's gatherings for more than ten years. I have also learned good skills in compassionate communication, conflict resolution and group facilitation, through living here at Tui. I am blessed to be in a loving relationship with Jim. We have been in partnership for thirteen years now and have an ongoing journey together that supports and deepens us into ourselves, each other, and the sacred realms of relationship. Compost, hands in the earth, growing and eating food produced on our land, are things I love. I have now extended into becoming a smalltime farmer raising meat for the community. I'm enjoying learning about the incredible mysteries of the soil, the relationship between the Universe and the Earth, and how they influence plants and us.

The Tui Community nestles into three valleys next to the Abel Tasman National Park and the pristine estuary and beach of Wainui Bay. This well established intentional community has a unique culture built on a strong foundational belief in the sacredness of all life and developed through consensus decision making in weekly community meetings, the deep process of the heart sharing circle, the importance of emotional clearing and conscious relationship, while living in harmony with the land. Established as an educational trust, Tui opens its doors to hundreds of international visitors each year who come seeking "something more". Jim and Suzi participated in the co-creation of the men's, women's and co-gender gatherings and these too, established unique cultures of their own, combining immersion in nature with deep process, sacred play and ritual, drumming and shamanic practices. I was privileged to be part of the core group in a women's gathering when staying at Tui in 1996 and I found it to be an intensely powerful experience. The group became a container for an archetypal healing energy which I intuited to be profound and far-reaching in its effect. The gatherings have built an extended community throughout New Zealand and beyond. Jim and Suzi have now further extended this healing culture and community, into much needed, ground breaking rites of passage work with teenage boys and girls, in their Tracks and Tides programmes. I approached this interview eager to discover more about how this very distinctive culture has evolved and to honour the important work that Jim and Suzi have set in motion.

All views expressed here by Jim, Suzi, or me, are simply our views and do not reflect the Tui Community as a whole.

**Rose:** Let's start with what it means to you to live your passion.

**Jim:** My passion connects me every day to the moment, to what's going on, and the more there can be a connection to every moment of my life, the better I feel. When I'm feeling good and I'm moving in a positive direction, the better the resonance in my everyday life. I am a person who can get passionate about things. As I look back through my life, I can see the passions I've held along the way. They've not necessarily all been golden passions, good social passions; there have been shadow passions as well, but they've always been passions that have involved people.

I was tremendously caught up with soccer at London University, which is a huge federal university with about 40,000 students and about twenty different colleges. We had a football league which consisted of sixty-five teams and I ended up overseeing that and overseeing the university programme for six years too. Then through my profession as a dentist, which was happening to me along the way, I found I didn't like to inflict pain on people and so I became passionate about using alternative delivery systems for dentistry, using intravenous and inhalational analgesics and so on, in order to be able to serve people in a more comfortable way. That was in South Africa in the '70's. I stopped playing soccer there and published in international research, travelled a bit through Europe doing presentations about these particular IV techniques around a particular drug, which is still used today. I seemed to have an inherent connection to serving people and helping people with their life situations.

I then went on from there to become extremely passionate about dentistry. I had an epiphany when some American dentists came over and I learned about preventive dentistry, biological dentistry, ecological dentistry, and became absolutely impassioned with that. Alongside me, was Cherrie, and we were in partnership professionally as well as personally. We decided to move to the best place in the world we knew of for dentistry and that was North America. Over a period of years, we developed a huge, very alternative style of practice there, which was turning over a million dollars a year.

Another aspect I'm aware of, when I think about my passions is, often they're a bit off the wall and I end up being offside sometimes with conventional society and having run-ins with organisations that supposedly govern our society. It's never been a big thing, but being in opposition to professional practice ethics, for example, and looking at other ways of doing things, has definitely been a passion.

**Rose:** Is it through being an innovator you've found yourself in conflicts?

**Jim:** I've certainly been influenced by, and fascinated by, people who see things a bit differently: artists and alternative thinkers, outrageous colourful people. I think it's a desire on my part to be a more colourful character; yet not being particularly creatively talented, I seem to have found myself in a place of providing forums for other people to find themselves, and as I do that, I find myself in those places too. Certainly,

I feel myself to be a leader, not always a confident leader, but my leadership has developed in the last few years as I've become more settled in myself. I'm a team person too, I like doing things together with others, and the deeper the process the better.

Finally, we decided to sell up everything in North America and look for the next thing. Finding Tui community in '89 was certainly a serendipitous thing.

**Rose:** Had Tui been going for several years by then?

**Jim:** About five or six years, so we weren't there right at the beginning. Tui provided the environment for more of my passions to blossom. Soon after we arrived here, I had a major process in my life when my relationship with Cherrie came unglued after twenty-six years. Huge prolonged processes around that eventually led me to find my way into men's work, as a resource for support, and for comforting myself and finding reassurance in the stories of other men.

**Rose:** That must have been pretty early on in the men's movement?

**Jim:** It was right at the beginning. In fact the men's movement here began the same year it officially started in the North Island with Rex McCann. There had been some mutterings with groups starting in the '80's, but nothing continuous.

**Rose:** Did you bring a group together or did you join a group that was already going?

**Jim:** I went to a men's leadership gathering at Tauhara, one of the first ones, met men up there and was amazed by it. I was deeply in my process around the breakup with Cherrie and the men's movement became a very important aspect of my life. I found challenge, reassurance and excitement with the colourful nature of it, particularly with the outdoor wilderness style. Then my mentor, Michael Jude, who was touring through New Zealand, showed up in the Bay and gave a presentation based on North American Indian practices. The interesting thing was, just before I'd left Canada in the late 80's, I'd had a couple of years of intense involvement with a shamanic initiation process over there and I had a North American Indian shamanic initiation, albeit quite an alternative one. It wasn't about going to live with the tribe; it was run by psychiatrists who were investigating ways of shifting the psyche by using the vehicle of the North American Indian traditions. Now, here was a Cherokee pipe carrier in Golden Bay and we had this resonance! The next thing, we were doing an outdoor wilderness gathering here!

**Rose:** It sounds all very serendipitous.

**Jim:** Very serendipitous. There's part of me that's an inherent networker. I don't like the word networker, but I like connecting people and talking: "Oh, you're doing that and you're doing that! Look at this! Let's get together!" So I started connecting the men's gathering work in the North Island with what we were doing down here. The next thing was to challenge the women to start up their gatherings. Then the idea was for the men and women to come together, as we did at the end of the first few gatherings. That was the beginning of the men's and women's gatherings! They went on for five or six years in that way and were deeply a part of the community growth in those

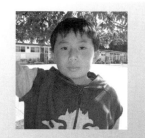

*Mark: A Joy Seed*

My WHOLE NEW WORLD seed would be a joy seed that grows into a joy tree. The joy tree would spread joy with its beauty. It will grow into a world of peace and simplicity.

days. A lot of other work was going on as well. Many people were into Domain Shift, so that was influential, and the community process was very big too. We engaged with all these different currents as a real, on-the-ground living process, living those relationship interactions as we went along. That had something to do with the potency of the evolution at that time.

**Rose:** As you're talking, I can see the threads that became, to my mind at least, quite distinctly Tui culture: the outdoor, wilderness aspect; the shamanic aspect; deep processing and emotional clearing; relationship work; learning how to be a community and make community decisions. A unique set of threads came together, almost accidently it seems.

**Jim:** It fell out of the community style of living, as you know from having been here. The community meetings are huge teachers, talking and interacting around the stuff of life. Along the way we learn very useful skills and it's only when you go out from here, you find that you understand. I say you, because you came here Rose and were really involved with our process and with the gatherings. It's an everyday training in relationship, which the outside world doesn't have as a resource.

**Rose**: I see it as a real service, something quite unique and powerful you offer to all your many visitors. I've never come across anything quite like it.

**Jim:** The men's gatherings grew and I went off to different parts of New Zealand and different parts of the world, like South Africa, Canada and America, to wilderness gatherings, along the same lines as those we were doing here. At the same time, we had a host of kids here. At one stage, we probably had fifteen to twenty teenagers living here. It was an intense learning time! Suzi and I were very much a part of saying to the kids: "Ok, rather than just fighting with the community, why don't we start a series of meetings for you guys?" So we started to do that and they came up to the house. It was mayhem some of the time! It represented a confrontation between the more conventional side of the community, who wanted a pretty straight way of raising the kids, and the other side, which was quite strongly alternative. Later, there was a very good and serviceable turning point that happened between those different aspects.

The kids used to come up here, and they could invite whichever adults they wanted and if they didn't want adults, they could say no to inviting them. They gradually became empowered and we started doing events for the kids called "A Movable Feast", a designer event where we went out to the west coast. It was actually an *unmovable* feast, although the original idea was to have caravans, tents and so on, and go from one area to another. Once we had the kitchen set up, one of the primary tenets was they could eat whatever they wanted, whenever they wanted, at any time. We'd go out to the west coast and hang out there for a few days then some of the parents would come and visit. Some would be along for the whole thing, but the kids had the right to call it as they wanted it. It empowered them to bring their issues back into community meetings and stand their ground. They were a very active tribe.

**Rose**: What motivated you personally to do that work?

**Jim:** The fact we were stuck right in the middle of it and had five boys! *Laughter.*

**Rose:** That's a good enough reason!

**Suzi:** Our house seemed to be the centre of a lot of the activity. Jim and I realized the community house wasn't the place where the teenagers could hang out. There wasn't actually anywhere they could go and just play music when they wanted to and cook meat and all those things teenagers do. So we consciously opened our house up to them as a place where they could just be together with some pretty clear agreements.

**Rose:** They must have felt safe with you?

**Suzi**: They felt safe and I think by offering the house we got their respect. In fact, they were great, because there were times when it was all too much and we'd say: "You just have to go" and they'd go. There were other members of the community who thought we were sucking up to them and not being clear with our boundaries and letting them get away with things. They were at those teenage years of experimentation around alcohol and drugs and we had the general feeling that actually, we'd much prefer they did that here where we could see them, rather than going twenty minutes into town and us having no idea what was going on. There was a general agreement in the community amongst the adults that it was our preference to create safe and very clear parameters for that.

**Rose:** Your house is very much in the middle of the community, isn't it? I admired you being right there in the middle with everything happening around you. That must have had its challenges at times?

**Suzi:** Ooh, it had a lot of challenges, particularly coming home when we were both dreaming of a quiet night and we'd drive into the car park, to hear the boom, boom, boom of the music and we'd think,

"Oh my God, that's coming from our house!" We'd walk in the door and the whole house was covered in kids! I don't know if you were here at the time we put the tipi up behind the house?

**Jim:** We decided we'd move out, because they had this amazing ability just to hang out and be in each other's company. They had a huge personal growth workshop continually going on. Although they were in resistance to what was happening in the community, they were certainly observing and resonating in their relationships. You'd hear: "Well Crystal and Zora, you don't seem to be getting on very well. I really think you should sit together and have a facilitator and talk this through." They were conflict resolving and going in and out of quite deep intimate relationships with each other within the group. There was a huge learning process going on which was absolutely marvelous.

To complete my part of the story, I was passionate about the men's movement and developing this aspect of the relationship between men of all different ages. Because of what was happening in the community, I wanted to have younger men to our events. I always managed to get some younger men, eighteen, nineteen and twenty year olds, to the men's events, against some opposition I have to say, because most of the men in the men's movement at that time and it may still be so, were men at midlife crisis, who wanted to talk about what terrible times they had with their fathers.

**Rose:** They were there for therapeutic reasons?

**Jim:** Yes, a lot of the focus, probably more than half of the time, was spent on the midlife story of men and how that was evoked; I was in that midlife thing too, early fifties. Anyway, the idea of mentoring came up in the men's group and I had the idea of conscious mentoring and invited all the men I knew who were interested in conscious mentoring to a workshop. That concept still holds good for me to this day.

A mentor is someone who is chosen, and to be chosen and to be of service, he needs to make himself attractive to the people whom he would like to mentor. Men love to be chosen to teach and to be alongside young people.

I met the caretaker of some land up in the Marlborough Sounds in a men's group in Nelson. He lived at the old post office on the point, on three thousand acres of land, which you could only get to by boat. He wanted to take some time out, so I said: "Why don't I take it on? I'd love to bring the boys up and that will give you a break." He would come and deliver us to the woolshed, which had an outdoor kitchen, and our time was spent around hunting and fishing. We'd take five or six boys and five or six men, with the men being consciously aware they were being invited along to get alongside the boys. We visited there over the full moon every month for the best part of the year and there was a huge learning process with that. It was a powerful time! The caretaker, who was a pig hunter and had these wonderful big bull mastiffs he'd trained, was having so much fun with us being around on the property, he actually became a part of the group! Early in the morning, the boys would go off into the bush pig hunting with the dogs, some of us would go deer hunting, and some fishing. We'd get back to camp about lunch time and the rule was you had to eat something of everything you killed.

**Rose:** Were they mostly young men from Tui or were others included by that time?

**Jim:** It was put on for the young men of Tui, but there were one or two boys from outside, sons of a few of the men from the men's gathering, as well as the five or six boys from Tui.

**Rose**: Why do you think both the men's work and the young men's work are so important?

**Jim:** I'd have to backtrack to why Cherrie and I left North America in the first place. We had a fourteen year old and a six year old and were frustrated by the style of life we had there. We were worried about the school system, drugs, fast cars and so forth, and the huge materialism we were involved with. We were class one yuppies with all sorts of money, all sorts of toys, boats, property, and all the rest of it. We went through a big shift there in realizing the value of having good friends around, who our kids could learn from, and we knew that would be reinforced in community, where, by definition, you're rubbing up against people all the time.

**Rose**: So it was a choice to deepen life experience for yourselves and your sons?

**Jim:** It was about actually unpacking and unfolding that relationship aspect between the older and the younger men. A person can have a huge amount of talent and skills, but unless they consciously choose to offer those skills and offer to teach those skills, then no progress is made, as far as I'm concerned. It's nice they can make their beautiful wooden widgets and they're great artists, but nobody learns from that. It was about confronting myself and other men and saying: "Hey! Make a decision! Be proactive! These young people are all around. Get alongside them! They actually do want to talk to you! It might not seem like it, but they are dying to ask you questions and learn from you!" This is how Tracks is to this very day. Men are told their primary purpose for being at an event is to be themselves, tell their stories and get alongside the kids.

There's always a men's group of about fifteen to eighteen men in the Tracks events. They're willing to offer themselves as mentors and become fathers, uncles and facilitators in training. I want them to get hold of the idea that part of their job, as I see it, is to learn how to be a good influence on society through mentoring young people and, of course, that can be cross-gender.

There's a ritual where men from the men's group stand up and go to the centre of the circle, then sit down around the fire. Everybody else is around the outside: the home-group leaders, the directors, the new boys, the trackers (the boys who come back a second time). Then, the men who are proposing to be mentors are asked to stand up and the coaching is to learn how to describe themselves, who they are and what they have to offer, in terms a thirteen or fourteen year old can hear. A lot of men will go off about: "I'm really a good solid honest man and I like to sit down and have deep discussions." But this doesn't really appeal to a thirteen year old! The men then stand up and do their "dance of the conscious mentor" and eventually all of the men have presented themselves. It's quite a quick process. We try and get them to be precise. We end up with a dozen or so mentors standing up around the fire, with their backs to the fire, and the new boys are asked to go and choose a mentor. They wander around and go shopping; it's a quiet process. Then they each stand beside a man. Sometimes a man will get one, two or even three boys choosing him, three is the limit. Sometimes, a man won't get chosen at all. Then we ask the boys to describe why they chose who they did and we ask the men to describe how it felt to be chosen, or how it felt to be not chosen.

Men are hugely honoured by being asked. There's a deep part of them that really wants to be in service to the next generation. Our task in the training is to get them really aware of that and for them to go away motivated to do more of that.

**Rose**: What a beautiful process! It's also really beautiful the way it's unfolded for you: starting with your looking for something for yourself, to being very active in the men's movement, to working with the younger boys and men and then going into Tracks and training mentors.

**Jim:** Yes, Suzi and I have our five boys and my elder son Jay is living in the house with us now. He's very involved in Tracks and we do a ritual called "the father separation" which is an individuation process. The father stands at one side of the circle with the son standing on the other side connected by a string which they hold across the fire as they talk to each other. There's a facilitator for each pair: "Ok Jim, this is your son Jay. Do you have a few words to say to him at this time? Are you willing to allow him to step into the next stage of his life?" Often the boy's father isn't there, so we get a surrogate man to step into the father role. Then we say to the boy: "This is your father sitting over here. Do you have a few words to say to him at this time, and are you ready to step into the next stage of your life?" Sometimes they aren't, but mostly they are. And then they burn the string! It's a symbolic thing. I've been doing that with Jay every few months for the last six years now and every time we do it, there's a significant shift. It brings up emotion in me. At our last ritual, he had become a father and as a consequence, I am now a grandfather!

**Rose:** Congratulations! I feel really touched by that, Jim.

**Jim:** The most thrilling part for me, Rose, has been to confront this misconception society has, that young people are essentially egocentric. The myth is men are essentially egocentric, boys definitely, and especially teenage boys, are the most egocentric beings on the planet. The truth is, when you take that boy through a process where he now becomes a young man, and he's valued and recognized by his community and honoured, and you invite him back to the event as a young leader, what we call a tracker, to help the next lot of new boys to come through; in other words, you put him into a servant leadership role, he is so there with his heart! They come from their hearts! It's brilliant! It's amazing how much they want to help! That, for me, has torn apart one of the dominant myths of our society.

**Rose:** That's a very important truth to put out into the world.

**Jim:** I think so. If you get boys into heart, they are brilliant, beautiful, loving creatures.

**Rose**: That's so good to hear, Jim. This is such important work! Is it open to anybody?

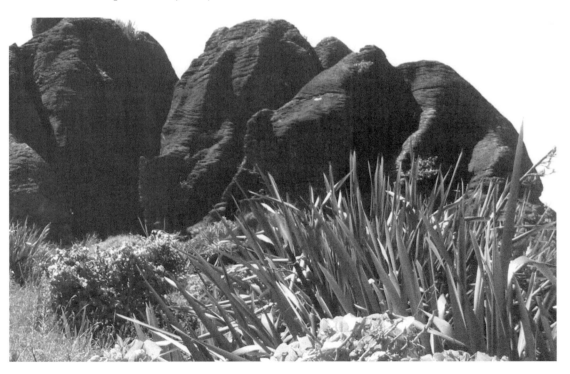

**Jim**: We're working with thirteen to fifteen year olds, but we have boys come back as young leaders, so they can still be coming back at seventeen or so. There are no restrictions. We're essentially a preventive programme. We're not looking to work with delinquent youth. Everybody wants a weekend process that will take a supposedly rotten kid and turn him right around and bring him back as a sweet sociable person. We prefer to take normal kids and really build their self esteem, honour their spirit, and help them on their path. It's touching when you see a boy in the first day or so and you look in his eye and say: "How are you doing?" His eyes are looking around and he's wary, saying: "Where's it coming from? Where's the put down?" Of course, we have to train our trackers to shift gears. We say: "This is not about you this time. This is all about the new boys and this is how we want you to get alongside them." It's all about friendship and getting them on board, enabling them to feel accepted and seen. If they're frightened they're held, and if they're noisy, they're still held.

**Rose:** Thanks, Jim. Suzi, do you want to start at the beginning again and tell me what it means to you to live your passion?

**Suzi:** I guess my passion is what I carry with me, it's what I move into this world with, depending where my interest is, or what's happening in my life. Before this, it wasn't work I was passionate about, instead it was being a passionate parent or passionately growing vegetables. Maybe my passion is being a midwife, not in the conventional sense, but more in the sense of raising seedlings, whether they're kids or plants or whatever, and helping them to grow to their full potential.

**Rose:** Sounds like a very fulfilling thing to do.

**Suzi:** Passion's a word I like because it can cover many things: gardening, my love for little babies, and it also comes into Tides. My excitement about Tides, and my hope is, we are supporting and empowering young women to go out into the world and be fully themselves.

**Rose:** Since I've known you, you were the gardening coordinator for a while, then really into art, and I know you ran a vegetarian restaurant at one time. Of course, you were very involved with the women's gatherings too. It seems to me whatever you do you get really passionate about it!

**Suzi:** That's right, when I look back at my life, it hasn't been one thing necessarily but whatever it is I'm doing, I carry it really passionately. Then something else comes along. There are so many things I love and am passionate about, sometimes I have to let some of them go for a while. For example, right now Tides is my main focus, so I have to let go of my art. I always find it a bit of a struggle to let things go and not try to do it all.

**Rose:** A difficult balance when you're living in community, I believe.

**Suzi:** One of the biggest things I'm learning here is how to maintain my own equilibrium whilst being in community.

**Rose:** Do you think you've cracked that one?

**Suzi:** I *have* cracked that one and the community itself is having a bit of a change and rebirth! We're in a stage of chaos, and I quite like chaos because I think from it can come wonderful growth. Some people aren't happy being in chaos. They're afraid we might never get out of it, or might end up going somewhere they don't particularly want to go. But I think chaos is healthy. With the women's gatherings, we could guarantee the third day would be chaotic. It happens in Tides too; the moment where everything becomes a bit shaky, is usually the day of our transition, which is the main ritual on the third day. It's amazing how often something completely unexpected happens that day.

**Rose:** You don't have difficulty maintaining yourself in chaos?

**Suzi:** I notice I can get a bit tense and anxious and want to help contain it, but I'm more relaxed about it now, because I think it's a natural place. Initially, I think a lot of people respond to chaos as something out of control, which they don't want. I believe it's a necessary and important part of the process of change.

**Rose:** Yes, and that's relevant for where we are globally too.

**Suzi:** It will get more chaotic and then something new will come out of it. What's really helped me is, we've been involved here with Gabrielle Roth's "Five Rhythms", and chaos is an important stage of the cycle. After the chaos, comes the lyrical. It's helped me to come to terms with chaos and understand it doesn't have to be just out of control; it can also be really grounded.

**Rose:** What do you think are the necessary skills for maintaining yourself in chaos?

**Suzi:** I guess trust and knowing it is ok to be there; trust and acceptance. I'm fortunate being a pretty grounded person. I imagine for some less grounded people, there's a more scary aspect.

**Rose**: Let's talk about the women's gatherings: I know you were very central to them for several years.

**Suzi**: I was part of the core group and I really enjoyed the excitement of holding the gathering with a group of women friends, whom I valued. We always had an understanding: regardless of whoever showed up, we'd be there for each other! I really enjoyed that!

**Rose:** Is the importance of the core group to hold the energy and embody the culture?

**Suzi:** Yes and the core group changes every year as you know.

**Rose:** My experience of being there with you as part of the core group was wonderful! In fact that gathering was the most powerful group experience I've ever had.

**Suzi:** Those initial gatherings were incredible, particularly when we were meeting the men on the beach at the end. After a time, the core group got a bit stuck. The same things were happening over and over. We became stale and it wasn't refreshing any more. Then Jim started Tracks and suddenly there was another way for some of us to move on which took us to a new level: from the service of self to the service of others. My excitement with Tides is that we are there to help these young women come through to empowerment.

Tides is about becoming more aware of the importance of conscious rites of passage, from birth through to death. The rite from girl to young woman is quite major. Talking with a group of women about how we celebrated this, we realized most of us hadn't had any celebration and actually we found it quite a difficult, awkward time! Maybe if we had held some conscious marking of that transition, it could have helped us to move into becoming women more easily.

**Rose:** Threads of self were left behind because there wasn't a significant ritual to mark the passage from girl to woman?

**Suzi:** No one was there to tell, show, or guide us, into how to be a young woman. Tides is blessed by having Tracks, two years ahead of us, paving the way. A lot of our programme is similar to theirs; we have the two rituals Jim mentioned, the father and the mentor process, which we put into our own context. We meet down in the tree field for a four night, five day event for thirteen to sixteen year olds, and we too, have young leaders who come back to help the new girls coming through. I don't necessarily see all the girls who have been through, some of them fall away, but with the ones who do come back as young leaders, it surprises me how many of them make a shift by coming through Tides. We also establish a relationship with parents and talk with them and the girls about the move into adulthood, and how wanting more freedom requires more responsibility. Beforehand, we say to the parents: "When your daughter comes back, maybe it's a good time to renegotiate agreements and look at how you can have a win-win situation rather than the tug and pull which often seems to happen." We encourage negotiation and shared responsibility and it amazes me how many parents come back and say: "It's so good what's happening with our daughter."

**Rose:** It seems a core group is really necessary to hold the culture. I'm sure you bring the distinctive Tui culture into Tides?

**Suzi:** Yes, if you came to Tides it would be very familiar. A lot of the culture and how we hold our circles come from Tui and from the women's gatherings, with a bit more intentionality and focus for younger people.

**Rose:** I bet the young women absolutely love it! It must be so empowering for them. I have two more questions for you, Suzi. I'm sure you must have learned heaps and developed many leadership qualities through doing this work. Could you reflect a little on your time of being at Tui, your involvement with the gatherings and what you've learned?

**Suzi:** I think my skill is in midwifery. I'm very good at getting behind people and supporting them. My strength isn't necessarily standing up at the front. Leaders play different roles and I'm a space holder, a guider and very much a supporter. I have learned heaps at Tui about how to hold and facilitate groups, and I took that into the women's gatherings and increased my knowledge and learning there, particularly how to hold and carry people in process. Then once again, through Tides, I'm learning a great deal and a lot of that is around things I never expected, particularly through stepping into the role of coordinator. There are certain issues like child abuse, for which I have to learn the legalities. For instance, if we have disclosures of any form of abuse, what do I do? Like any gathering, we have an agreement of confidentiality but, when we're dealing with young people under a certain age, we have the responsibility if we hear something that is endangering them, to report it. I'm learning hugely all about that.

**Rose:** This brings you more in touch with the society at large?

**Suzi:** It does, and it's something I'm enjoying. Tides is bringing me into more contact with the community workers and we're working more together. They're supporting us and sponsoring girls to come to Tides.

**Rose:** It's very encouraging and exciting hearing how this has all evolved. It's quite special. One last question: I see a new conscious culture emerging in New Zealand and I'm interested in how a new culture develops. It seems to me, over a period of twenty years, the Tui community has developed a very distinctive culture. Does that feel true to you?

**Suzi:** To a certain extent, yes. I've just been to a training session with community workers and there's a movement from the government around nonviolence. They're looking at family violence because it's so extreme here in New Zealand and how a more respectful and accepting culture can be incorporated into all institutions that have relationships with families and children. They're looking at violence in the widest sense you can imagine and how to introduce concepts and practices of nonviolence to youth, to create a culture of nonviolence amongst them. I came away with a lot of pride, because I believe this is what's happening at Tracks and Tides. The nonviolent culture is right there! Some of the things we're introducing and helping these young people to develop are respect for self, acceptance of each other, and a more compassionate way of relating to each other.

**Jim**: I think Suzi's put her finger right on it! Girls are much more articulate at that age, while teenage boys need another way of approaching each other and new communication skills as an alternative to the macho style and attitude. The premise we use in Tracks is "seeing, calling, and acknowledging." We use a generic ritual to learn the skills of deciding to look at somebody in an observing way and "seeing" who they are. It doesn't take very long. You need only know them for an hour or two to see their essential aspects. Deciding to "call" is to approach and speak to that person in a positive way. Then "acknowledging" is deciding to learn the skills of honouring and blessing. There's a large part of Tracks which is centred round the ritual of celebration, with a beginning, middle and an end. In the honouring and acknowledging, a thrill comes through these boys when they are seen by a group of men who value them and tell them: "I really like the way you do that." It has to be in their language. We have to learn how to speak their language, so we can be heard. A lot of adults don't speak children's language, especially with boys. Boys don't have very good communication skills, but they have huge listening skills. They're hearing everything, and if they hear bullshit, they'll turn off right then. But if they hear a genuine wanting to communicate with them, they'll open up.

**Suzi:** For me, the culture of change comes through the role modeling in Tides and Tracks. It's really important to have a good, solid group of same sex parents who can honour and respect the teenagers. The language is compassionate, empathic, clear, and honest. There's no right and wrong, no judgements because of what you're wearing or not wearing. We're really trying to create more acceptance. Both Tides and Tracks provide training for the women and men who come along to the events; they're coached how to be with these girls and boys.

**Jim**: I think the enemy to our young people and to our society is stereotyped advertising. Literally thousands of images come at them every day, indicating they should be this way or that way; whatever the advertisers choose for them. The bare midriff teenager, that's their uniform, a little bit of shiny in their navel. It's boring, but they're so looking to identify with what's supposed to be ok. What we're trying to do is say: "Hey! Actually, it's deeper than that! You are inherently a wonderful person and you are a seed! You're germinating! You're flowering! You're unfolding! Just look at you! Look at how you move! Look at how you laugh! Look at what good company you are! How clear you are in your speaking!

We're looking to find those things that are real and genuine within a huge energetic forum. We have a group of forty men plus, of all different generations. There are usually about eight or nine new boys and throughout the whole event, all of us, are totally, constantly, looking to frame everything we do, to be able to be heard and felt by those boys. You can see it! On the first night they arrive, after they've been on a six or seven hour walk and we're all standing in the darkness at nine thirty at night; the boys are there and the men are there, I always stand up and say: "Hey! Get this! You maybe won't believe this for a day or two, but we are all here for you! All we men are here because you're important and I'm going to remind you about this." After a day or two I look in the eye of even the most doubting boy and say: "Are we making it with you?" And you can tell by the way he looks back at you, by his behaviour, by the way he is. He responds: "Holy mackerel! These people are here for me! They're here for me!!!" Suddenly they realize they're of huge value.

I think boys and girls in society are undervalued. They undervalue themselves and it doesn't help that their whole culture is so stereotyped. They become fearful and confused and they need deeply to be valued. In indigenous cultures, the African Masai culture, for example, they understand that at a stage of life, there's a redness growing inside, it's the fire, the "litimo" growing inside the child, and it's incredibly important to allow that to work. Young people need to feel held and I don't think they feel held in our society.

**Suzi:** No, they're really not.

**Jim:** The world's a scary place. All these expectations are scary.

**Rose:** I can hear just how passionately you want to reach them. It's beautiful! Thank you both so much for your work.

*We shall dance for the unborn, for the children*
*We shall dance for the unborn, for the children*
*Dance the dance for the unborn*
*Dance the dance for the children*
*Dance the dance for the unborn*
*Dance the dance for the children*

# *Vivienne Anne Wright*
## Kids love Peace

Vivienne is a "Citizen of the World", currently resident in New Zealand. For many years Vivienne worked in advertising, specialising in creative writing and Cause-Related Marketing, whilst living in a house full of other people's children. Born in Australia, beneath the mountains and beside the sea in sunny North Queensland, Vivienne has lived, travelled and worked around the world, including a lengthy sojourn on a lush tropical island in the Gulf of Siam, where she built a home without walls and a glorious garden. She is Founder and Executive Trustee of One People One Planet, a registered Charitable Trust with a mission to bring together the children of the world in mutual harmony and respect, to work together in a child-focused, child-driven manner towards a sustainably more peaceful world. Vivienne is also founder of New Horizons Unlimited and leads spiritual journeys in her spare time. www.onepeopleoneplanet.org

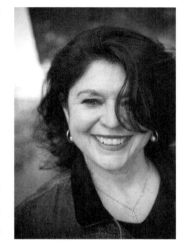

**Vivienne**: Living my passion defines my life. To attempt to live fully and passionately, it seems to me we need to be sure what it is we are most passionate about and work towards empowering that purpose.

In my life, circumstances and opportunities have coalesced to mean that right now I am in a place where my elemental desire is to know I'm making a difference at a time when the planet is at a pivotal stage in its evolution. I look into the future with a great deal of optimism. I believe we can achieve much if we come together on a commonly agreed platform of respect and sharing and work together towards a commonly agreed goal. It is time to find new ways of living together in harmony, with the greater good of all, our major objective. For me, this translates into being part of the formation of a process that works towards leaving a legacy of connectedness and mutual respect for future generations, in any way I can.

For many years I have been entranced by one of Gandhi's most famous statements: "If there is to be peace in the world, we must place it in the hands of the children "

**Rose:** You live your passion through leading the wonderful global peace project, One People One Planet?

**Vivienne**: Yes. I believe our children have the potential to create a better future, especially if we grant them the opportunity to come together across the boundaries of time and distance, to share their views, their aspirations, and their fears. That's what my life is focused on now. Previously my greatest joy and possibly the fundamental building blocks of my life as it is now, were living in, and developing communities in other places, globally. I have been blessed with uncommon opportunities, all of which have led me to the realization that my greatest desire is, in my lifetime, we will all be carrying passports saying: "Citizen of the World, currently resident in New Zealand" (or wherever any of us may call home.)

**Rose:** Yes, to be a true global citizen is something to aspire to! You've been nurturing this project for four years now?

**Vivienne:** Four going on five years.

**Rose:** Tell me how it started?

## *Seeds of big dreams born out of crisis*

**Vivienne:** Peace has always been my passion. Kids have always been my passion. These two elements came together in a flash of inspiration, very powerfully, when my life was unexpectedly riven apart. It was an incredibly challenging, traumatic time. Everything that had previously been the anchor or the structure of my life, the picture and the shape of a life I cherished, was taken from me. I had built my home and my life on an island in the Gulf of Siam, in Thailand and with no warning, no money and no job I ended up back in New Zealand. In response to this, and with a great deal of generous support from loving friends, I took time out to come to terms with my new status, to reflect and to understand the deeper meaning of events and the unexpected gifts that could come from this.

I set about planning a positive way forward into a new life and a new future. I was aware I needed to move beyond my small world of pain and loss, and dream big. I knew I wanted a life that would be, in my terms "big, bright, bold, and beautiful". So, the process I embarked upon was to allow myself a time of retreat to go deep within. I came out of that process, thinking I had been granted an incredible opportunity to begin again and to live in a purposeful, meaningful way, committed to something I really believed in, larger than self. I came to the conclusion that the way to mend my hurting heart was to realize my gift to the world. That realization in hand, three questions emerged: What can I do – what shall my gift be? What is it I really feel strongly about and passionately connected to? What are the gifts and talents I can bring to bear, that are meaningful and useful? The answers came over a period of intense reflection. When I really focused on what I most believed in and wanted to work with, it became clear it was all about working towards a more peaceful world, the world our kids are going to inherit.

Like so many others, I am deeply concerned about the world we are leaving for our children. What are we doing with our mindlessness and our separateness? How can we start to see each other as a brother or a sister with a different skin colour or a different language? I can see what we most need is a new way forward. I can be part of that! I can dedicate myself to that!

**Rose:** It seems a greater sense of meaning came to you from a personal crisis? That's so often the way it happens, isn't it? Crisis, and the loss of something or someone we love, is a doorway to a deeper life purpose.

> *Liam:*
> *A Seed of Remembrance*
>
> *I would like to plant a seed of remembrance and everyone would remember and be wise, like teleporting and telepathy instead of cars and computers. If we remembered who we are then it would not be hard to do this. There would not be computers or cars or pollution, and people would be able to talk to every living thing on the planet.*

**Vivienne:** We are taught the deeper meaning of crisis is opportunity for change. For me, things were brought to a burning point by the crisis. In a situation like mine, in which I was badly betrayed and lost people and things that gave my life meaning, I had to take it higher, to a bigger place. To begin again, I focused on elements I've always felt strongly about.

Over many years, I've chosen to live in different communities around the world and have gained a great deal in terms of life skills, cultural diversity, and a dream for a much finer future, if we could all come together as a global, rather than merely a local community. This was the opportunity to put some of those dreams into practice.

**Rose:** You chose something big. A BIG global project! I'm impressed you seized the opportunity to transcend a situation of deep grief and transform it into something so hopeful for the future. That's real Love-in-action!

**Vivienne**: It came to me quite strongly. I made the commitment my life would be well lived and worth something ultimately meaningful in the larger sense and I would spend a period of time in definite service to a higher ideal or philosophy. Over a period of four to six weeks, I began developing the concept and the name. It looked and felt good and at that juncture, I began seeking input and support. At the outset, I took the working concept to my lawyer and said: "Now you've got me through my personal trauma, I think I need a registered charitable trust!" He made time for coffee and we went through the concept together and he said: "This is the most amazing concept I've ever heard and I think it will work, we must do this, and I'm in! "He was the first other trustee. From the day I put it in front of the first person, it was taken up very strongly, and that's been part of the story. Immediately following his involvement, I put the idea in front of three other beloved colleagues from my 'past life' as director of an advertising agency. All of them were excited, all of them said "Yes!" And from the outset, to this day, they are involved respectively as Chairperson of the Board, Head of the Advisory Group and trustee.

We have unbelievable support from community leaders, kids, educators, specialists and consultants. The project has grown with other people's input exponentially. It's developed an extraordinary life of its own, fueled by the enthusiasm and support of a wide range of visionary and luminary supporters, whom we have consulted and been enriched by. It just keeps developing in size, vigour and scope, harnessing new and emergent technological advancements and knowledge, as we progress. It has its own life and its own path, as any idea which has come into its time does, I imagine. It's incredibly exciting and life enriching.

## A global project for peace consciousness

**Rose:** You're developing a very creative project for global peace consciousness, focused on empowering kids and connecting them around the world, and in the process, you're getting lots of adults involved as well!

**Vivienne:** Developing peace consciousness, from our point of view, is a practical idea and project. It's based on the fact that what we share with others is simply the desire to be liked, understood and respected, and this shared desire is far greater than anything that divides us. The kids just get it! The kids are extraordinary! The thought of being able to join in global community excites them, especially when we make it clear they will be consulted as we progress.

As a group, we are committed to not only developing it, but putting it in front of the kids, to ensure all we prepare and manage for them is focused on their needs and desires. We have been delighted with their enthusiasm, uptake and emerging concepts for further development. They get it and they want it! It's an idea and an opportunity we can't ignore at this pivotal time in the evolution of life on Earth.

What most excites us is that the children are able to communicate their dreams and concerns clearly. We've been pleasurably amazed by how sophisticated they can be about articulating their dreams and their desire to come together. This drives my commitment to give them the forum and support them to create community that is for kids, by kids, with kids; with future developments focused on their input and needs.

We're going to maintain an as-safe-as-possible, secure-as-possible, ICT platform for the kids to form alliances that will ensure for the first time ever, they can work towards having a real chance to talk, learn and develop together, negating boundaries of time, distance and culture. We know they will develop a world view and a global community, defined by them; a place that has no imposed ideological agenda. We'll be encouraging them to feel free to explore their commonality learn to respect and celebrate their differences, and have fun being Peace Pals; the name they have chosen for themselves.

**Rose:** I love the way you're supporting children's autonomy!

**Vivienne:** Yes, and that commitment is so central to our core philosophy and they're so ready for it. We're focusing initially on five to twelve year old children. I always ask when it comes time to talk to the children, that the Principal and teachers merely introduce me and allow me time with the kids. I like to gauge their interest and their understanding of our organization and its purpose, based on the name One People One Planet, and the knowledge it is for them. And Rose, it takes them about ten minutes! They consult together, and then every time they come up with the fact, it's an organization for kids to communicate with each other, to become friends all around the world, utilizing computers. It is quite amazing and very satisfying. A very, very typical response is one I got from a little Maori boy at a school here in Auckland, who just looked at me and said, "Does this mean I can have a friend in Afghanistan?" And I said, "Yes, Syrhan, you could. In fact, we have a trustee in Afghanistan at the moment, so it's really interesting you've picked there. But in the beginning, it might be email only, until we've defined what their technology is. Is that ok? " He replied, "That's seriously hot stuff, Miss!" I responded, "So I guess you think that's a pretty cool idea?" He just looked at me and said, "If we could be friends, we wouldn't fight and there would be no more wars, and we would share the food and nobody would starve. Do you get that, Miss? "And I said, "Yeah, that's the idea." Then he said, "Kids love peace, Miss!" It was an incredibly beautiful moment. This kid had been hit so badly his arm was broken and yet this was his private world view! We've registered "Kids Love Peace" as a domain name. They came up with the name Peace Pals, because that's what they want to be. Our travelling Internet portal is called a Planet Mobile and the kids think that's really cool.

**Rose:** So, you're aiming to build a global community of empowered kids!

## Launching Peace Pals

**Vivienne:** The One People One Planet premise is based on building a global community of kids, to give them a presence and a voice on the world stage, a chance to shape their own future. We launch this year with our first live global connection of children working and talking together about peace. The launch project is called "Peace Pals: Children Connecting for Peace". Every aspect of our proposed projects goes past the kids and they endorse it. Any resources provided for the kids to work with, or learn from, will be in response to their request. We have already had some indications of what they want and will ask for, and we're thrilled to see the sort of thinking the kids are already employing in their projects. They are entirely congruent with our core operating principle.

One of our management board members had an epiphany one night, when he suddenly sat forward and said, "This is what it is in really simple terms. There'll be a ten or twelve year old in Levin and he or she'll connect with a ten or twelve year old in Pakistan. Our kid will grow up to be the Deputy Prime Minister, the other kid will end up being a Governor of the Reserve Bank or something, and over the years, they'll have formed a strong friendship and there will be communication and commerce between the two countries." And that's it! The forging of lasting alliances, building respect, trust and commonality and shaping their future! I feel it's an honour and a privilege to be part of an evolving opportunity for children to shape the world.

**Rose:** What a wonderfully timely idea! A kid's movement for peace, supported and serviced by adults.

**Vivienne:** As adults, we have to accept that our role and responsibility now is reduced to that of stewards and guardians, that our time has passed, and we need to be placing the future where it belongs, into the hands of our kids and future generations. I think it was the Hopi Indians who always made decisions seven generations out. I want the kids to get that concept. Our experience and our research show us clearly that they're more than capable of getting that!

**Rose:** It's all so essentially simple. I particularly love the emphasis you place on the involvement of the children. Yet I know you've worked very hard to involve many adults too.

## Creating a national and global community of interest

**Vivienne:** Yes we have made some amazing connections along the way. Fantastic people! We have been blessed by the enthusiasm and very substantial support of a wide range of community leaders, specialists and consultants in many fields. We would not be where we are today without the support of some very fine individuals. In fact, some time ago we were granted an audience with, and have received the written endorsement of, His Holiness the Dalai Lama. This was an extraordinary experience, a huge blessing and a real milestone for us.

**Rose:** That certainly is a great blessing! The Dalai Lama is such a wonderful ambassador of peace.

**Vivienne:** His Holiness is almost universally recognized and honoured as one of the greatest advocates of peace ever. He blesses our endeavour, which we as an organisation treasure. The audience with him was a high point in our development. In fact, his endorsement will form an important element when it is read in full during our launch event. Our idea brings out the best in people and almost without exception, everyone we have approached has joined us and given the best of their abilities, wholeheartedly. It seems when I look back and around me at the wonderful people that surround and support us, the most common response has been "what can I do to help?" We have an enormous following and support network of many hundreds of people, many of them very well known and respected in their area of expertise.

This network is growing all the time, as we develop the organization and the projects. This is exemplified by "Peace Pals: Children Connecting for Peace". This project has widespread support from the Mayors of two of New Zealand's biggest cities, both of which are Peace Cities (Christchurch and Waitakere City), schools in New Zealand, the highly respected Global Mayors for Peace, the Mayor of Hiroshima, schools in Japan, principals and teachers, including the Apple Distinguished Educators network, and hundreds of kids! Children in schools in Auckland, Christchurch and Hiroshima are working on a platform paper, that's been put together by the Associate Principal of an involved school, a wonderful woman who is highly regarded by her peers. It's been tracked and evaluated in each participating school by Professor Ken Ryber's Action Research, after which an academic overview will be overseen by a Professor at Waikato University, who's in charge of the e-learning research function there. That's a project going global and live, which will be monitored every step of the way, so we can chart interest, involvement, development, change, and future projects.

We have the launch being filmed and a dvd being prepared, and the launch will be screened on the Ministry of Education's Virtual Learning Network, into primary and intermediate schools throughout New Zealand. Many hundreds of people are involved in this one event alone. It is quite breathtaking and very satisfying.

In this project, the kids are defining how they respond in their own creative way and the process is being filmed as they work within their own group at school. Then they'll come together on a half day hui (gathering), connecting kids in Auckland, Christchurch and Japan. The kids plan on filming themselves presenting their projects on the day, as well as during the process at school. We'll compile it all onto a dvd, which will include the formal research overview and statement about what these projects do. Then we'll have living proof of concept, so when we go to someone and say we would really appreciate your involvement and your financial support, we can present them with the dvd of the children speaking live. It will give a compelling idea of what we do, what the children do, what they're telling us and what they want.

We have been invited to attend an education sector annual conference in February next year, which will comprise the top one thousand ICT teachers and principals in New Zealand. This will be a wonderful forum for raising peace consciousness through the dvd. One of the suggestions is that we put together a classroom of kids at the conference, and have them working on a live global project, so teachers from nonaligned schools can observe the kids, their enthusiasm for the projects they develop, and the value and worth of One People One Planet for the kids, and ultimately for society at large.

**Rose:** It all sounds so well thought through, well organized and well supported, I'm quite amazed you've had difficulty getting funding.

**Vivienne**: It's a bit of a mystery to us why it has taken so long for us to achieve funding. Everything we've achieved to date we have self funded, or we've been gifted support in terms of people's academic qualifications or their ability to help us develop a concept, or just provide man or woman power. We've made funding applications to organisations and trusts we would have thought would be highly receptive, and the most common response is: "Come back to us when you've got runs on the board." There is limited funding in the not-for-profit sector. It is understandable potential funders would be cautious and practice a high level of due diligence, but we would genuinely welcome that, and be entirely transparent and accountable. We're a fully registered charitable trust, with the requisite Board of Trustees, Management Board and an Advisory Group. In each segment, we have specialists and consultants who are leaders in their field or specialty, including education, internet safety, research, technology, peace studies, global communication, community building, governance, public relations and branding.

It is hard to get fully operational, with an established base of operations and staff, when that is the prevalent attitude. We need startup capital to fund the ongoing development of our ICT platform to ensure it is, and remains, cutting edge. Also administration funds, so we can begin the journey into a high level of self sufficiency. Somebody's got to be first to give us funds to get fully underway.

I do sometimes wonder… this idea is so well received, why can't we get it funded and happening faster? For example, we have a principal in one of our schools who is a Baccalaureate Principal and he can link us with colleagues in Kosovo, China, Thailand and Turkey. We've been blessed by Imam in Kashmir to take it to the schools there. We have schools waiting in Calcutta and Nepal, good links in Pakistan, and we have someone in Cambodia saying: "Bring it here; I have an orphanage of one hundred kids and a computer lab. Let's get started!" A trustee who is currently working in Afghanistan plans to contact an incredible American who has founded fifty schools in Afghanistan and Pakistan, where peace is a major element in the curriculum. We also have the opportunity of working with the Apple Distinguished Educators, about seven hundred strong, spread around the globe. The Distinguished Educators here in New Zealand are already involved and are saying: "We can just roll it out through our network and build clusters around it. We can make this happen!"

Yet we just don't have the funds to be able to do that immediately. It's frustrating to be struggling with limited resources with the opportunities we have in hand, with an idea as well received. We'd love to be in a position to utilize all the resources we have, backed by adequate funding, to be able to have everything in place, to let it go and have the kids involved everywhere we have links and opportunities.

**Rose:** I wish you luck with the funding! I hear your frustration at not being able to run with everything you've put in place to take it to its full potential. I know funding is a challenge for so many people who are working for a better world and that can be such a drain on one's creative energy. One of the things that impress me about this project is how multidisciplinary it is. You've drawn together support from so many different fields. This, in itself, is a great success and rich resource. It's a co-creative community, especially remarkable when so many eminent people are being drawn together to promote global peace consciousness. This is a testament to your own goodwill and determination, and to the goodwill of everyone else involved. You also have so much participation happening with kids, even without funding!

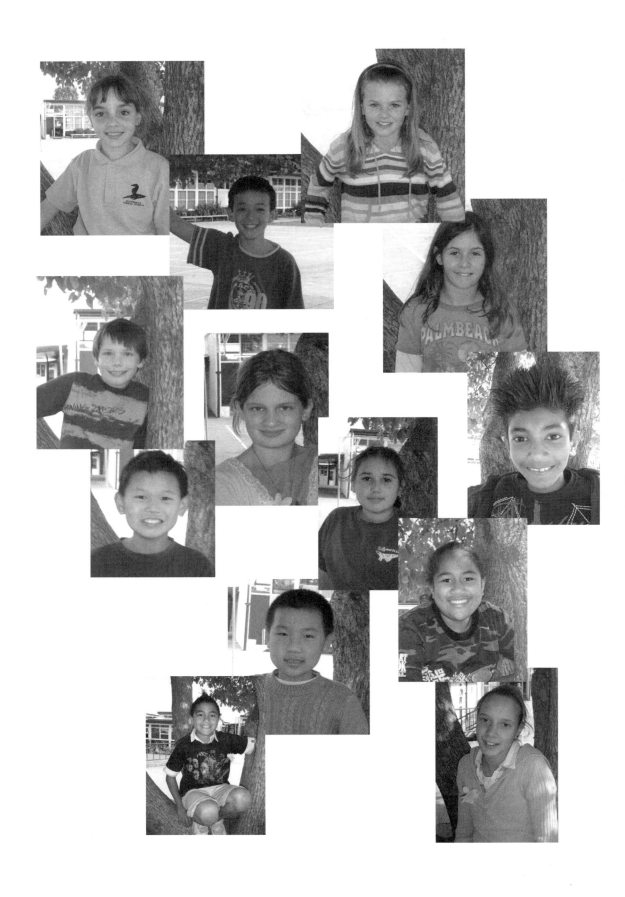

## Show casing New Zealand expertise

**Vivienne:** Yes, there are other projects going on independently in various schools around the country. We have children developing a website, which will be incorporated into our formal website, which is being developed by a senior lecturer at the Manakau Institute of Technology School of Communications. We have children writing haikus, making dvds, presentations and writings of all sorts. Each participating school encourages its kids to come up with individual projects, which align with our mission and purpose. This is a great way of checking that the concept works with kids, measuring their enthusiasm and involvement, and watching how they develop their concepts, values and ideas. We are committed to maintaining an ongoing research component to evaluate progress and ensure we can develop it, as the children want it, including as fast as children want it. We're going to have to harness current and future technologies for this to work; obviously this commitment to ongoing technological development means the One People One Planet ICT platform is also going to showcase New Zealand expertise, which is another fantastic thing!

**Rose:** This project has gathered a lot of momentum, I'm sure it's going to fly! How are you different now from when you started out four or five years ago? You must have learned so much and it must have been very challenging for you in many ways being the catalyst and holding such a big project.

**Vivienne:** It's been incredibly challenging and very, very fulfilling. My life is now hugely different and I would not have it any other way. I feel blessed. Along the way we have been, and continue to be exposed to new ideas and developments and wonderful, visionary people in all walks of life. In truth, it has forced me into a way of life that's very focused, in some aspects, it hasn't been easy to live, but it has always been developmental and fulfilling. This is what I'm doing full time and I live hand-to-mouth, which is a challenge. The more we've gotten into it, the more we have appreciated that peace consciousness is a practical project and an idea whose time has come. Even more than difficult or challenging, it's been illuminating and exciting. Every day brings fresh challenges, but whenever I'm talking to the kids, or in the schools, I get hit anew with the realization of just how powerful our concept is, realizing how ready and capable our children are to be "Change Agents of Peace" and just where they're going to take it as soon as they're given the opportunity.

**Rose:** It sounds as though everything is in place and ready to go! You've had to be very determined over a sustained period of time to achieve that!

**Vivienne**: Yes. It is, however, much more than a personal achievement. A dedicated group of highly motivated and commercially experienced professionals has come together, bonded by the vision of what we can empower the kids to achieve and to share. We've worked hard together and we have all really put ourselves on the line for this. It won't be my personal achievement when we achieve our aims. It has been a major combined effort and it will be a shared achievement. The day we launch "Peace Pals: Children Connecting for Peace" it will be a significant milestone and I am sure we'll party!

**Rose:** How do children see the world we're living in? Are they aware of the global crisis?

**Vivienne**: They're amazingly sophisticated; they talk about wars, poverty, fighting, misuse of resources and destruction of the planet's species. They talk about it being not fair. They talk about feeling scared. They're worried about the sort of world they're going to inherit. They're aware things could be a whole lot better and how important it is for people to talk to each other and be friends with each other and share. Those are the words they use. It's really exciting when you spend time with the kids and have the opportunity to hear what they want and what they would do to change things for the better, if they could.

Initially we're working with five to twelve year olds, but the next stage will be eleven to fifteen, and then fifteen to eighteen. The eleven to fifteen year old group is going to be really fascinating because this is where we will start to see the emergent leaders. We'll need to find a non elitist way to identify them and to offer them any opportunity we can to empower themselves, to take strong roles in the formation of their own communities.

The One People One Planet platform will have a plethora of activities and projects up and running at any one time, generated by the kids and supported wherever and however we can. We're already starting work on the next major project we'll set in front of the kids to do. Preliminary research has indicated it will be enthusiastically received and develop into a huge, multidimensional and global "kids voice for peace". From that point on, we hope the kids will define their own projects, once we've got them up and running, with the idea of what they can do for themselves. This next planned project is very, very focused on a creative opportunity for the kids to voice their dreams and their desires for peace in a highly visible and fun way.

## *A common purpose and vision*

As a group, we have a common purpose and vision which empowers us to give One People One Planet all we have and all it needs. We all know in our hearts this is a powerful idea whose time has come and we all want our lives to count for something. We have proved to our own satisfaction that, by empowering the kids to form their own global community, within a generation or two, they will have had the means to create a sustainably more peaceful world. The only way to do that is to put it into the hands of the kids because it's their future. That's what keeps me burning bright.

We work on with the adult agenda of raising money, and developing the ICT platform, and formalising the arrangements with the schools, knowing this is for the greater good and it's going to bring kids together across the boundaries of nationalism, race, creed and gender.

Children of all persuasions will come together in peace, to talk peace and to know the pathway to enduring peace is practicing peace in all things. We have a motto: "Peace is the pathway to Peace" and we all live it in everything we do with One People One Planet. We have found that it builds a very solid and sustainable culture for our organization, so you see, we are learning too as we go.

The children are already talking about being brothers and sisters on the planet, respecting and learning to celebrate and enjoy their differences, to find ways to become friends and learn to share resources. Beginning with the younger ones, we'll get them at a time when they have the least prejudice and give them an opportunity to explore all of this. Fabulous!

**Rose:** This is a truly wonderful and optimistic vision, Vivienne. Where did the seed come from initially?

**Vivienne**: To be true, I owe a debt of gratitude to my parents and their ethics and world view. My father passed away recently and it is a sad loss in my life. His life was dedicated, in no small way, to enriching the community he lived in and I know he would be proud to see what we are achieving with One People One Planet. My mother has always been an enthusiastic and tireless supporter, and I am blessed with special friends who understand my passion and who support me hugely. New Zealand has a reputation for taking a lead in matters of global significance: the atom was split here, the vote for women first started here, we are leaders in nuclear disarmament issues. We have a history that encompasses many areas in which New Zealand has led the way and I think this is one of the next ones, a new stepping stone into a much brighter future.

It feels like all the things I ever did in my life came together in this: all the experience, the expertise, the enthusiasm for a new way forward, became the underpinning of the initial idea. All the time I was living overseas, experiencing different cultures, the seed was growing within me. It was enriched in the early days of our evolution by spending time (with Dominique LaPierre, the internationally recognized author of "City of Joy" and philanthropist, and his wife Dominique) in leper ghettos in Calcutta. I saw children of the very poor so determined to go to school and be educated, as I worked and lived with some wonderful Catholic priests called the Prada Brotherhood in Calcutta, who have dedicated their lives to educating the poorest of the poor.

These kids walked kilometres to school and then kilometres back in the afternoon, to work to support their families. I close my eyes and I can see their little bright shiny faces at desks just wanting to learn! These kids remain a symbol. If we can just provide the means, the children will learn and develop together, and devise a new way forward into a brighter, safer future.

## From New Zealand to the World

Although One People One Planet is based in New Zealand, it is an emergent global organisation, which focuses on empowering the children to move forward together into a sustainably more peaceful future. I know from experience, many people would do something altruistic, if they could only find something meaningful to do. We welcome involvement. This is an opportunity for people to support, be part of and help us to grow this idea.

**Rose:** I'm glad to hear the kids are aware of what is happening in the world and have so much desire to do something positive.

**Vivienne**: It's amazing what they come up with. I've said to a couple of principals and teachers, "Lord bless me! I didn't expect them to be so sophisticated or articulate." And they just laugh. There's a great school here with a multicultural roll of kids including Maori, Polynesian and Asian and they have won an international reputation for their podcasts. I was sitting talking to their ICT teacher, a wonderful woman who is widely recognized for the amazing things she and her colleagues are working up with the kids at their school, and I remarked: "This might sound patronising, or as though I just didn't know, but I am so amazed at the kids' enthusiasm and uptake and their desire for what we're offering." She looked at me, smiled widely and said: "They're ready for this. They know the world is going to be theirs and they want it to be a better place." This school has done fantastic things with our projects.

We're not the first organisation to focus on kids and peace, but we have found an innovative, creative way to do it, which makes the most of the technology of our times. There was an organization called STEPS founded about ten years ago by a teacher here in New Zealand, based around the nuclear threat. So ten or twelve years ago, they realized the kids have a role to play. We're not the first, we're not the pioneers in the concept, we're just pioneering a project that's a world first, that will be global. It is New Zealand based! It is about peace! Here we go again! Wave the flag for the Kiwis!

**Rose**: Yes! May it spread like wildfire!

## Post-Script

PEACE PALS: Children Connecting for Peace, the first live global project, was launched on October 8 at Waitakere City Council Chambers, hosted by His Worship the Mayor, Bob Harvey. Waitakere City is New Zealand's newest Peace City in the growing global network.

Over one hundred and twenty children (Peace Pals), representatives of the schools involved in New Zealand and Japan, came together in a live video link, to share their ideas and desire for friendship not defined by cultural, political, religious or gender issues. The kids laughed, talked and shared their hopes and dreams for a peaceful world as they presented the projects they had developed, based on the project designer, Barbara Dysart's platform paper. It was an extraordinary and heartwarming event – the first of many. Amogh, an Indian boy living in New Zealand, exemplified the day and the potential of what we have begun together with his statement:

"On the outside we might look different – we might sound different ... BUT INSIDE WE ARE ALL THE SAME"

Here are some comments by involved teachers and children:

**Barbara Dysart, DipTB.ED, Associate Principal, Summerland Primary School, Auckland** (Project Designer: "PEACE PALS: Children Connecting for Peace")

There are a number of reasons for listening to children. These include moral and practical reasons. Listening to children is common sense as they can often shed light on a topic an adult can overlook. Children are not so blinkered by differences that may exist, such as race or religion. They can give valuable feedback and have a lot to teach us about the world and its problems. For these reasons alone, we need to listen to children and their perceptions of the problems and issues they experience.

**Jenny Sinclair, Teacher, Kaiapoi Borough School, Christchurch**

Participating in One People One Planet has encouraged my students to explore, question and construct their own moral framework in which to view their world, now and in the future. They are constantly asking: "Are we making a difference?" Integral to their ongoing commitment to rethinking is the real connecting to real people available through One People One Planet. Today's children are the citizens of tomorrow. Their future is being made today! They inherit a very different world, full of pressing issues that come straight into their homes each night. The pro-active approach through One People One Planet, gives a human face to the issues and they are gaining a sense of actively partic-ipating in making a better future. The opportunity to actively make decisions and see their ideas come to life has an enormous impact on their motivation to learn and to see that learning links to action. They are so passionate about being listened to and One People One Planet has been great in allowing them to tap into authentic concerns and learning. The contribution they are making through this involvement has had a positive impact on self-esteem and they are beginning to understand that we need to accommodate different world views. Kids are awesome!

**Harrison:** "Being a part of this allows us to have our say. In the news, everything is negative, we feel smothered and they only mention the good things once. It would be better if we focused on the positives."

**Kayla:** "Normally adults don't listen. They think we want stuff for ourselves but we're not selfish. We are impacting the Earth and animals are becoming extinct every single day, we have to do something about it before it's too late! If we had a peaceful planet maybe everyone would be able to listen to each other."

**Jarred:** "If we had a peaceful planet we would be able to sleep at night and not worry about even little things. Justice would be important. "

**Taige:** "People realize what they are doing to our planet and they see the effect it has but they continue being selfish. We have to be responsible and start making the right choices."

**James:** "There are lots of things to worry about such as weather patterns and poverty. Kids actually worry a lot about the world. We shouldn't have to worry about so much! But if we have good ideas, then they should be listened to."

**Jessica:** "If everyone remembered that the things we do affect each other, we would be kinder. I think it's important to be kind to animals too. If you are kind to animals you are kind to people."

**Sarah:** "When we work with the little kids we help them with their emotional intelligence, even when we don't mean to, it just happens because we are helping. I think everyone needs to be kind. "

**Stephen Gordon, (B.Ed., M.A.), Assistant Principal, Sunnybrae Normal Primary School, Auckland.** The One People One Planet project has been an interesting and valuable experience. The approach is student-driven; students not only decide what question or statement they wish to respond to, but also how they will respond: with a picture, written response or podcast, for example. The teacher supplies the question or statement and guides from the side. I have been impressed by the deep thinking and the responses give me hope for the future.

**Vikki Rihari, (Diploma Teaching, B.Ed. (Teaching), Teacher, Henderson North Primary School, Auckland.** When I presented the One People One Planet project to my class, I began by talking to them about the impact war has on the world. Many of the children were very knowledgeable about the awful things that come from war and couldn't understand why people couldn't just get along and talk. I then introduced the concept behind One People One Planet and explained that we had been asked to share our ideas about peace with the rest of the world and to help develop One People One Planet from a children's point of view. The children were in a buzz at the mere thought that they could have a voice - and maybe someone would listen. It was a great learning experience for them to think about how they could change the world and what would happen if we could all just get along. As a result of the project, the children have been kinder and caring towards each other, which has been a great outcome for me as the teacher. If more schools could get on board, and the media became more interested and involved, then I think this project could develop into something enormous and incredibly valuable socially.

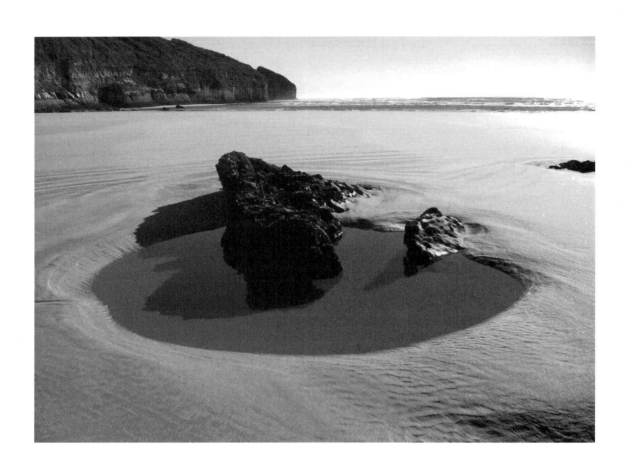

# Conclusion

## Towards a globally responsible world view

*What does it mean to live your passion?*

*How does living your passion become Love-in-action?*

*How does Love-in-action seed a whole new world?*

All the people included in this book are living their passion and expressing their creativity, each in their own unique way. They are authentic people who refuse to compromise their integrity and do their best to stay aligned with universal values, working for the good of humanity, holding a big picture global vision, and "bringing the vision down" by grounding it in local contexts and specific focused projects.

There is positive energy and an uplifting presence in such people. They engender a sense of empowerment. Their way of being and what they're accomplishing support me to turn my attention away from what is not working and instead focus all my energies on creating from my own vision and passion. When a group of authentic people come together to co-create, there can be a synergy which lifts and moves everyone into the creative flow. A resonant thought field forms, which enables ideas and concepts to be communicated very quickly, over time and distance. The influence of social innovations undertaken in a spirit of conscious awareness, and in alignment with universal principles, should not be underestimated. It only takes a few people to seed new ideas and when these ideas are seen to work, they quickly become mainstream.

With authenticity comes the realization of the essential interconnectedness of all life: all living beings exist as part of one interconnected, interdependent and ecologically balanced whole. This realization carries with it a responsibility. Once we have realized our essential interconnection, we must be in service to it. There is no going back to a dream of mere personal salvation. This understanding of the essential unity of all Life is now embraced by science as well as by ancient spiritual traditions and cultures. As the global crisis hits home, more and more people are waking up to this essential truth.

A globally responsible world view is crucial if we are to survive as a species. This begins within each individual and grows into an openness to embrace and celebrate difference and diversity and to serve the greater whole. In other words, individual responsibility and autonomy are the foundation for co-creative community and a peaceful, global culture. This book has endeavoured to show how individuals acting on their heartfelt convictions can, and do, make a difference.

For many people in the world, any sense of cultural belonging has been lost or destroyed. We live increasingly in a world in which people from different cultures live together side by side, yet cultural differences are effaced by the "dumbing down" of consumerism and the mass media, resulting in a bland monoculture of bare survival. This may give rise to a wariness of the concept of global responsibility, as people confuse it with the enslavement of globalisation as it has been created by the power hungry and self interested minority. Or else, the problems in the world appear so overwhelming that retreat into resignation or despair is seen as the only option.

Ken Wilber warns: "People are not going to expand their present views or outlooks by much more than 5% at any given time. So if you are trying to push a very big picture at them, they are probably going to shut down, and might get angry and then start calling you names."

I, along with others in this book, may be out-of-line with consensus reality, but we're choosing to maintain faith in the ability and willingness of the human spirit to rise to the challenge before us, difficult though it is. This faith is not an idealistic wish or hope, but based upon practical solutions and innovations already coming into being, as people connect with each other to share creative ideas, resources and mutual support.

The vision for humanity emerging from these interviews is growing from the grassroots. It is a vision of local and global interconnectedness, based on an understanding the world has sufficient resources to sustain everyone if we live simply, in harmony with nature, sharing what we have and working together.

What is obvious from these conversations is that personal and social transformation do not grow just from ideas, but arise from a foundation of a daily consciousness practice and a philosophy of life evolved and brought to maturity over years, through a willingness to go on learning and acquiring new skills.

Developing the skills for real community and co-creativity is not easy. I believe it is our greatest challenge as a species. Creating projects and taking action are relatively easy; really listening to each other and appreciating each other's differences are not. Sharing leadership and resources is a challenge for most people. Going beyond our prejudices and assumptions, opening our minds and hearts to each other, taking the time to discover whether we do in fact have shared meanings for the words we use, learning to value each and every person for their unique contribution, this is love-in-action.

Personal autonomy, mutual acceptance and the celebration of differences are the foundation on which to build co-creative communities. From here, it is then possible to reach out and forge creative alliances around common evolutionary goals, to service and support peace consciousness, true education and global networks. Healthy autonomy is nourished by identification with something bigger than self: cultural roots, a connection to the land, a sense of belonging in community, and being at home in humanity, Earth, and Cosmos. How will we preserve the wisdom and knowledge of our diverse cultures and languages, as we learn to live harmoniously together?

## A new story for New Zealand

This book is based on the premise that at this transitional time, nations can grow beyond purely national interest to global responsibility by identifying and acting upon their "new story". What has emerged in these pages, I believe, is a new story for New Zealand. It's a story of passionate, soulful initiative and servant leadership, with the potential for role modeling a whole, new, nonviolent culture to the world. Can we imagine and dream it into being?

Other nations have their own emerging stories too. I wonder what the new story for the United States will be, or for the UK, South Africa, Iraq or China? Stories which reach into the future and point to a higher calling for a country can unite people behind a positive vision. I believe the nourishment many people are hungering for is hope, inspiration, meaning and a sense of purpose derived from being empowered to make a positive contribution. Beyond the chaos, war and destruction, we have a new global story to co-invent and each of us has a part to play in how that story unfolds.

Distressed and disillusioned by the emptiness of globalised monoculture, more and more people are turning their backs on it, freeing themselves to create a new globally responsible culture, in line with the integral values of living fully from mind, body, soul, spirit, community service, and passion. This culture is growing from the grassroots, in local communities. Whether these are intentional communities, where people choose to live together around a common purpose or values, or co-creative work communities such as that being pioneered at Swanson Sanctuary; living and working in community provide the perfect seedbed from which to cultivate the necessary skills to take us forward into a peaceful and sustainable future. These are the skills spoken of in these interviews: nonviolent compassionate communication; servant leadership; holding core values and a guiding vision; bringing people together into safe forums for dialogue and addressing issues of social injustice.

Humanity is at a major transition point in its collective life. To complete this transition from psychological immaturity to maturity requires us to evolve into a state of global consciousness. What would a rite of passage for this transition be like?

There is an awakening to the reality that the world cannot sustain our profligate Western lifestyle and there's an urgent need for radical change. It is my heartfelt hope and intention this book will contribute to a bigger inquiry on transformational skills. Together we can learn the transformational skills we need. Alone we can accomplish only a little. Working together, sharing our gifts and talents and our different forms of wealth, we become drops that coalesce into a rising wave of transformation.

## *Opening up the sharing circle*

Here, at the end of my story, I'm opening up the sharing circle. For those who have never been to a sharing circle, imagine our group of twenty-five passionate innovators seated in a circle, speaking as they feel moved and listening attentively to others. Our voices weave into a final recap and "dreaming", pointing towards the values on which the new culture may be built.

## Ordinary people doing extraordinary things: Bob

"Much of my life has been a journey of discovering the ability of ordinary people to do extraordinary things, and although I think anyone on this planet is capable of this, somehow New Zealand has the energy, a magnetic field that's new and fresh and easier to access. That to me is good enough to give it the acknowledgement and the dignity as unique in the world. We can be teachers of wisdom, of mystery and of soul politics, of environmental truth and consciousness. We can wear the cloak of mana and carry the mantle of wise and good facilitators. I believe we are the inheritors of more than dreams and visions. We are able to resonate the past into the future, and that is the connection I want to pass on to future generations."

## Aligning with the soul's purpose: Rose

"The creative process is about bringing everything to essence, or as close to essence as one can, so anything which is not essential has to be let go. This leads to greater simplicity. It may be the simplicity of living with fewer possessions or less external "security". It can also be a simplicity which comes through a process of integrating what can be quite complex ideas or experiences into more inclusive wholes. So there's an emergence of greater complexity expressed as simplicity, or wholeness. There's a sense of being pushed to one's limits by a greater power and having to learn both the laws and the discipline of how to co-create with that. Part of the discipline is being willing to go beyond the "little me", the needs of the personality, self indulgences and attachments. It's a process of holding a very clear focus and surrendering at the same time. You have to care enough to be willing to put in considerable time and energy, and yet be unattached to outcomes and not take it all too personally. It's really an exercise in aligning the personality and ego with the soul's purpose, and the soul has very different values and priorities. In this sense I think living one's passion is about being a creative artist, whether the work of "art" is one's own life, a community project, or in this case, writing a book."

## *Appreciating every moment: Kat*

"Joy is about being present. Being really present in whatever I do. I lose joy when I'm striving, and then the process becomes heavy and doesn't flow. It's about really appreciating life, appreciating every moment, and realizing what an amazing opportunity it is to be part of this! Yes, it's not always easy, and there are challenges, but I'm surrounded by all these incredibly inspiring people. I guess I feel the joy when I lose the expectations. When I lose the expectations, and I'm really real with what is right now, how beautiful it is and how lucky I am! It's a deeper experience of life."

## *Healing the Earth: David*

"If the world does take on drastic changes, which it may and is doing, I feel I'm getting better and better at living in a way which is an example of living without compromise. I intend to participate in healing the Earth, so we can look to living here for a longer period of time. There's also for me a real inner preparation of learning to know myself in my eternal nature and remembering who I am."

## *Social networking on the web: Will*

"It's already happened! The new culture's been created and has been running for seven years now, since the first dot.com boom. In the last year or two, there's been a profound shift in how things are happening, a coming of age of what we call Web-2.0 and that's about social networking on the web."

## *Participating in abundance: Frank*

"The first principle of permaculture is to observe and interact. Interaction is the key. It can be little steps. It doesn't have to all happen in one day, but a little bit each day and you'll start to flow.

What matters is recognizing the true abundance and participating in that abundance."

## Mirroring our divine nature to one another: Jonathan

"One of the core principles in Huna is that we're divine beings and as divine beings, we have only one need: the need for a mirror. In my reality, this thing we call the world is that mirror. The degree to which I forget my true nature as a divine being and the degree to which I start thinking I'm something else, is the degree to which I will start making life-taking choices. In Huna, there's no right and wrong. No good and bad. There's simply that which is life-giving and that which is life-taking and if I make life-taking choices, the consequence of that will be painful to experience."

## Seeing difficulties as stepping stones: Mirjam

"That was a huge, huge shift for us, to actually consciously choose to see difficulties as opportunities, not as evidence we're incompatible. They're actually an invitation for us to grow, which means we don't see difficulties as threats; we see them really, truly, as stepping stones."

## Practicing nonviolence: Rudolf

"What I notice is that when difficulties arise through very habitual responses, where I want to change Mirjam, I am actually practicing a mild form of violence. The nonviolent approach would be to see that I'm part of the equation and to ask the question: in what way is this part of me? What is the part of me I don't like? This is both very empowering and respectful."

## Committing to a daily spiritual practice: John

My practice involves a study of spiritual texts and current enlightened writings, and a regular discipline like meditation, which for me, is a Yoga practice. It's not just yoga for the physical body. The practice is concerned with refining or training the mind and body, so they become vehicles for the soul. If I want to develop spiritually, I have to have rhythm in my life. I certainly need and respond to that. It's not just about putting aside work time and the need to make money, although that can be a spiritual practice too, but making time to do things that really nurture my Higher Self. The mind is trained to gradually get a perspective on what it is I really, really want, which is a sense of unity and peace of mind. Through the training and rhythmic living, I get a clearer and more focused perspective on what a spiritual practice really is."

## Expanding consciousness through witnessing and surrender: Orah

"The passing on of the desire for expanding consciousness now can happen more effectively through the hands, rather than just sitting. People who aren't meditators suddenly start witnessing. We've had people describe incredible unity experiences and huge epiphanies, right down to really simple stories like getting financial stuff sorted out without even trying. The power of Deeksha is huge! It makes the expansion of consciousness so much more accessible, especially if people are prepared enough and trusting enough to let us put our hands on their heads. With meditation there's still a control: "I'm doing this". With Deeksha, it implies some kind of surrender, and then you receive what it is you're ready to surrender to. It's really quite a beautiful process."

## Experiencing more and more joy and gratitude: Anahata

"Deeksha turns the process of life into an ongoing movie of realizations. You get to witness each thought, feeling, sensation and outward observation upclose and personal. It takes the dullness out and perks you into really acknowledging what is truly being presented to you on your buffet table of experiences. The more allowing you are, the more you see. All of life is simply about "seeing", until one day, you are de-clutched from the hold of mind and dawn into silent, still consciousness, experiencing the movement. Emotions and thoughts still arise, but they pass through like birds in flight and disappear effortlessly. Joy starts to build and evolves into your normal state, with bliss coming and going. Gratitude grows exponentially to be the only outward energy you want to express, and Life goes on!!!"

## Going with the flow: Donna

"I resonate to live in the flow and serve for the good of all. I find when I am living my passion I am calm within and feel much love, joy, peace and harmony everywhere, in everything. For me living my passion is about being heart-centred and not fear-controlled. At this moment in time the world is changing rapidly and it's important to be in the now, to let go of attachment, and go with the flow. In practical terms, that means allowing our creativity to flow without placing limits of when, where and how. We have found by creating conscious relationships, taking full responsibility for ourselves and co-creating in a way of respect for all living things, in mutual support and resource, we have surpassed what we thought was possible."

## Building sustainable housing for a more co-operative world: Robin

"Co-housing is self-created community by people who want to live in a more co-operative world. The co-housing itself is about social organisation. A group of people get together, talk about how they really want to live, then start the whole process and develop housing which is designed for intentional community, ensuring it also includes safety and privacy. To the co-housing model, I also added the other half of it for me: the environmentally sustainable building, design and energy."

## Nurturing grassroots leadership: Margaret

"Project Port Lyttelton is just one group in Lyttelton. A number of us have been talking and saying it's silly reinventing the wheel and duplicating things. We're only three thousand people. Why not work more together as a group? We're beginning to get a name in the City as those who trial new models of social cooperativeness. Wendy's been talking to the Ministry of Social Development and they're always looking for grassroots examples that are succeeding. I attended a meeting with seven or eight overseas experts in this field in Christchurch last week and it was so good to hear them talking about sustainability. Both Wendy and I were there and we felt good being able to say: "We're doing all this!" It was affirming. The discussion was about play, celebration, embedded leadership at a grassroots level."

## Handling the basics: James

"I have a very strong sense the current form of society as it's promoted on tv is not sustainable. It's in deep trouble and that's reflected in all kinds of dysfunctions in society and communities. My interest is to support and find ways people can come to a greater place of trust with each other, and in part involves all the practical things which relate to food, shelter and clothing. If we handle those basics, all sorts of other wonderful creative possibilities exist for us to explore also. We can meet those needs in a way that is very, very gentle on our environment and creates a very gentle footprint."

## Co-creating with spirit: Robina

"There's a point at which every individual and then the collective of individuals, take responsibility for a project and for their own learning, their own process, their own communication skills, and so on. You can actually pinpoint that moment from one day to the next, stand back, just giving a little bit of guidance here and there, as well as bringing in resource materials, such as particular books, then basically shift into an overseeing role and watch the whole thing unfold. At that moment, if it's done from a place of non ego attachment and service, a shift happens and another dimension emerges which is spirit-led. I just look at the signs and feel the energy, listen to spirit and follow the synergy and timing of everything. This quality of energy may shift my plans on a daily basis, even to what materials we need to build with that day."

### Controlling the mind: Daniel

"What I'm passionate about is teaching the Art of Living, which is all about experiencing Oneness through something very tangible, which is the breath. Having done a lot of personal growth in the past, I've seen that can take you to the emotions, but there's a point beyond that we need to go to. That's on a level of trying to control this incredible thing called the mind, which wanders about all over the place, trips us up and says "oh, that's all very well but…", making excuses for our own actions. To control the mind, on the level of the mind, is impossible, but through the breath, you can actually control it. It's like the string on the end of a kite. As you pull the string, which is the breath, it uplifts the kite and the same happens with the mind. The breath energises the body and gives us a strong sense of ourselves. I encourage everyone to learn how to breathe, to learn how to meditate; from this, you get a sense of yourself as you relate to other people."

### Mobilising against injustice: Leanne

"It's that tipping point, when a stage is reached, where things are clearly unfair, where human rights are being abused, when things have gotten so bad people will rebel and ask questions. Information is so much more readily available through the Internet and that's been hugely part of the shift to people being able to mobilise together quickly, globally, in reaction to something they don't want. The speed of being able to communicate globally affects how quickly people can decide to act, but there's just so, so much more that needs to be done!"

### Healing the past and moving on in new ways: Chris

"Maybe it's about being willing to look at doing things in new ways, rather than repeating the old stuff that isn't working. It's about testing and evolving, rather than accepting the status quo. For us, it's about sowing the seeds of positive transformation. And, it's about allowing us to sing together in different ways; appreciating the different layers and identities; recognizing the past still has a presence in today; understanding the effects of the past are still needing to be healed; and moving on in positive ways."

### Being free to meet our needs and find our own solutions in our own ways: Takawai

"To me the vision is both peoples (Maori and non-Maori) are able to achieve their dreams and their aspirations in their own way. They're not forced into each other's systems if those systems don't work for them. For example, Maori won't be forced into a Pakeha education system if we know this clearly doesn't work for them. (50% of Maori boys leave school with no qualifications). It will be a society where there are choices and options…We have a beautiful land here in New Zealand, people want to come and live here. We've clearly got something really, really good. I'd like to see us building a healthier society more accepting of difference and offering many choices and options. Underneath that, there's recognition everyone is the same. I reckon that's the secret."

### Intergenerational learning and service are mutually enriching: Jim

"A mentor is someone who is chosen, and to be chosen, and to be of service, he needs to make himself attractive to the people whom he would like to mentor. Men love to be chosen to teach and to be alongside young people. A person can have a huge amount of talent and skills but unless he consciously chooses to offer those skills and offers to teach those skills, no progress is made. Part of their job, as I see it, is to learn how to be a good influence on society through mentoring young people. Men are hugely honoured by being asked and there's a deep part of them that really wants to be in service to the next generation. Our task in the training is to encourage full awareness of their potential and for them to go away, wanting to do more."

### Freedom and responsibility grow together and negotiation creates win-win solutions: Suzi

"We talk with the girls and their parents about the move into adulthood and how wanting more freedom brings more responsibility. We talk particularly with the parents beforehand and say: 'When your daughter comes back, maybe it's a good time to renegotiate agreements, to look at how you can have a win-win situation rather than the tug and pull which often seems to occur. We encourage negotiation and shared responsibility."

## Creating forums for sharing dreams and resources: Vivienne

"We've been pleasurably amazed by how sophisticated children can be about articulating their dreams and their desire to come together. This drives my commitment to give them the forum and support them to create community that is for kids, by kids, with kids. For the first time ever they can work towards having a real chance to talk, learn and develop together. They're already talking about being brothers and sisters on the planet, respecting and learning to celebrate and enjoy their differences, to find ways to become friends and learn to share resources."

## A whole new world view: Woods

"I see the special folks in your book as living examples of a new world view, a new metaphysics. World problems are so sewn together; we can't go on supporting individual-centered cultures any longer. We need to become a world balancing the self and the other, which can integrate the individual with an equally important communal and collective life. Normally we take on societal ways of doing things and we find a niche within the current social fabric. The notion, we're here to evolve new societal forms rather than remain stuck with what doesn't work, is new and different. Most people don't really yet know how to do that. We're so used to falling back on the cultural givens into which we're born and being very defined and limited by its older structures. We embrace a lot of things we don't necessarily have to embrace, because we don't think we have a choice. What we truly need, of course, is a whole new wave of social arrangements freeing us of the confinement of these older ways of doing things. In my view, Rose, you have succeeded in these refreshingly candid, novel interviews to suggest the new culture is deeply infused with richer spiritual meaning, of which we've been so bereft in the old culture. That's so hopeful!"

This is the vision! Be the change you want to see in the world. Become more conscious. Choose nonviolence. Handle the basics. Become Love-in-action. Act local, think global. Form alliances and co-creative communities. Be kind to the Earth and all living beings. Enjoy!

And until we meet in the Whole New World may your seeds of passion grow effortlessly towards the light.

*All of those for whom authentic transformation has deeply unseated their souls must, I believe wrestle with the profound moral obligation to shout from the heart – perhaps quietly and gently, with tears of reluctance; perhaps with fierce fire and angry wisdom; perhaps with slow and careful analysis; perhaps by unshakable public example – but* **authenticity** *always and absolutely carries a* **demand** *and* **duty***: you must speak out to the best of your ability, and shake the spiritual tree, and shine your headlights into the eyes of the complacent. You must let that radical realization rumble through your veins and rattle those around you......You were allowed to see the truth under the agreement that you would communicate it to others (that is the ultimate meaning of the bodhisattva vow). You might be right in your communication and you might be wrong, but that doesn't matter....only by investing and speaking your truth with* **passion,** *can the truth, one way or another, finally penetrate the reluctance of the world. One Taste, The Journals of Ken Wilber*

# References

## Opening quotations

**A New Earth: Awakening to your Life's Purpose,** Eckhart Tolle, Dutton/ Penguin 2005

**The Isaiah Effect: Decoding the Lost Science of Prayer and Prophecy,** Gregg Braden, Three Rivers Press 2000.

**The Universe is a Green Dragon: A Cosmic Creation Story,** Brian Swimme, Bear and Company. 1984

**Blessed Unrest, How the Largest Movement in the World Came into Being and Why No One Saw it Coming.** Paul Hawken, Viking Press 2007

## The Interviews

### Rose Diamond and Woods Elliott

**Migration to the Heartland: a Soul Journey in Aotearoa.** Currently out of print. A second edition will be published by Rose Coloured Glasses in 2008

**I and Thou,** Martin Buber, Touchstone 1970 (originally published in 1937)

**Joseph Campbell,** renowned author and mythologist who coined the term "follow your bliss". His books include, **A Hero with a Thousand Faces, The Masks of God, Myths to Live By.**

**Tom Atlee,** Founder and Co-Director of **The Co-Intelligence Institute** and author of **The Tao of Democracy.** His work focuses on developing our capacities to live as a wise democracy and on transformational exploration www.co-intelligence.org

**Spiritual Emergency,** Stanislav Grof, Tarcher/Putnam 1989

See also. **The Stormy Search for the Self,** Christina and Stanislav Grof

**Eckhart Tolle,** author of **The Power of Now** www.eckharttolle.com

**Swami Beyondananda,** political satirist www.wakeuplaughing.com

**The Gathering: Return of the Whale Dreamers,** a powerful and beautiful award winning documentary film created by Kim Kindersley about the plight of the Earth and of humanity. www.whaledreamers.com

## Kat Burns

**Recommended by Kat:**

www.positiveelements.co.nz Business supporting the unfolding of human potential and creativity

www.zaadz.com An inspirational online community

www.andrewcohen.org Spiritual wisdom, co-creation and inspiration

www.bravishi.org Inspirational communication, coaching and courses

www.cwg.org **Conversations with God** trilogy, Neale Donald Walsch

www.zeitgeist.com A film which will change your view of the world.

www.xresultsfoundation.com An organization supporting conscious entre-preneurs and social enterprise

## Will Lau

**The Celestine Prophecy ,** James Redfield, Warner Books 1993

**Sri Sri Ravi Shankar,** spiritual leader and founder of **The Art of Living Foundation,** dedicated to teaching yoga, meditation, the art of breathing and global service. www.artofliving.org

**Recommended by Will:**

**How to Win Friends and Influence People,** Dale Carnegie

**Seven Habits of Highly Effective People,** Stephen Covey (business/self development)

**E-myth,** Michael Gerber (business)

**Re-Imagine,** Tom Peters (business)

**Get the Edge,** Anthony Robbins ( self development, audiobook)

**The One Minute Millionaire,** Robert Allen and Mark Victor Hansen (heart based wealth)

**Rich Dad, Poor Dad,** Robert Kiyosaki (wealth)

**Building Wealth,** Dolf de Roos (wealth)

**Web:** www.slashdot.com Tech news feed

www.dailytech.com – Tech news feed

www.digg.com – interesting news from the web

## Frank Cook

**The Secret Teachings of Plants: The Intelligence of the Heart in the Direct Perception of Nature,** Stephen Harrod Buhner, Bear and Company 2004

**Starhawk,** author and peace, environmental and global justice activist www.starhawk.org

**The Secret Life of Plants,** Peter Thompkins and Christopher Bird, Harper and Row 1973

**Susun Weed,** herbalist and author, women's health www.susunweed.com

**Schumacher College,** an international college for ecological studies, based in Devon, UK,

www.schumachercollege.org.uk

### We can change our minds

**The Secret,** a DVD exploring the universal law of attraction, created by
 Sandy Forster. **www.WildlyWealthy.com**

## Consciousness is the Transformational Catalyst

**Coming Back to Life: Practices to Reconnect our Lives, Our World,**
 Joanna Macy, New Society Publishers 1998
**The Eye of the I: From which nothing is hidden,** David Hawkins, Veritas
 Publishing 2001
**One Taste, The Journals of Ken Wilber,** Shambhala 1999
**The Ever Present Origin, Jean Gebser,** 1949/53

### John Massey

For further information about Earth-Spirit Nature Retreats and celebra-
 tions, www.tuitrust.co.nz For contact with John about courses/
 workshops, practical herbalism/Yoga retreats, yogaia@orcon.net.nz

### Mirjam Busch and Rudolph Jarosewitsch

**The Virtues Project, Linda Kavelin Popov, Dan Popov, John Kavelin,**
 The Family Virtues Guide, Penguin 1997, Family Virtues Cards, Virtues
 Reflection Cards, www.virtuesproject.com
**Speaking Peace,** Marshall Rosenberg, Sounds True 2003
**Non Violent Communication,** Marshall Rosenberg, PuddleDancer Press
 2005

### Jonathan

Jonathan's personal website is at www.jonathanevatt.com. He has a few
 hundred pages of writing published at www.feal.org (see the Articles
 and Blog sections). On these web sites are links to many other useful
 sites and sources of inspiration.

### When we link heart to heart

Imaginal cells: **"Conscious Evolution: Awakening the Power of our Social
 Potential",** Barbara Marx Hubbard, New World Library References

### Anahata and Orah Ishaya

**The Ishayas Ascension**: www.ishaya.org
**Deeksha:** www.onenessmovement.org www.onenessuniversity.org www.
 globaloneness.co.nz
**Fire the Grid:** www.firethegrid.com
**Unity:** www.ishwara.com

## Creating New Models

A Crude Awakening, www.crudeawkening.org

The Eleventh Hour, www.11thHourAction.com

1. From "Changing Consciousness: Exploring the Hidden Source of the Social, Political and Environmental Crises Facing our World." David Bohm and Mark Edwards, HarperSanFrancisco, 1991

2. John Hagelin, Director of the Global Union of Scientists for Peace, http://hagelin.org in an article in Shift magazine by the Institute of Noetic Sciences, June-August 2007 www.noetic.org and www.shifti-naction.com

## Daring Donna

**Eduardo Manoel Araujo:** author of "A Possible Dream - from a non-sustainable materialism to a holistic sustainable life"

**Swanson Sanctuary Projects:**

**The Great New Zealand Street Party** - connecting a nation - 23 February '08 www.streetparty.co.nz

**Rose Coloured Glasses** - an adventure in co-creation through publishing.

**Open Arted** - an experiential heart weaving of cocreation through art www.openarted.co.nz

**Caring Communities** - www.ccp.org.nz

**Positive Elements** - www.positiveelements.co.nz - A sustainable garden offering products of quality, created with respect for the environment and the dignity of workers and their communities.

**The NZ Happy Gardeners** - sharing knowledge and resources throughout NZ.

**Suju Juice Bar** - 37 Channery Street Auckland City

## Robin Allison

**Cohousing: A Contemporary Approach to Housing Ourselves**, Kathryn McCamant and Charles Durett, Ten Speed Press 1994.

**Heart Politics** and Tauhara Wananga: www.heartpolitics.net www.tauharacentre.org.nz

**Servant leadership**: Robert K. Greenleaf, www.greenleaf.org

**Other resources**: www.wiserearth.org a networking website run by the Natural Capital Institute.

## Margaret Jefferies

**"Imagine Chicago"** Bliss Brown, www.imaginechicago.com

### James Samuel
**Findhorn Foundation:** www.findhorn.org
**James' blog:** www.yesterdaysfuture.net
**Recommended by James**: www.transitiontowns.org

### Robina
**Grounding Vision—Empowering Culture: How to build & sustain community together. A Manual of Participatory Tools for Social Change Facilitators,** Robina McCurdy, Earthcare Education Aotearoa

### Daniel Batten
**The Artists Way: A Spiritual Path to Higher Creativity,** Julia Cameron, Tarcher/Putnam 1992
**The Art of Living Foundation,** created by Sri Sri Ravi Shankar, dedicated to teaching yoga, meditation, the art of breathing and global service. **www.artofliving.org**

### Leanne Holdsworth
**A New Generation of Business Leaders,** Leanne Holdsworth 2000
**The Caring Communities Project**: www.ccp.org.nz

### Extending Community through
### Creative Resourcing and Partnership Building

**Catherine Austin Fitts** Navigating toward a more financially intimate world. www.solari.com
**Living Economies Aotearoa/New Zealand** www.le.org.nz includes a great resource section.

## Culture Making
**The Universe is a Green Dragon**, **A Cosmic Creation Story**, Brian Swimme, Bear and Company, 1984.
**Awakening Faith in an Alternative Future,** Senge, Scharmer, Jaworski, Flowers

### Chris and Takawai Murphy
Hinewirangi Kohu: **Broken Chant Poems**, Rosemary Kohu and Robert de Roo, The Tauranga Moana Press 1983/84
**Screaming Moko,** Hinewirangi Kohu: the Tauranga Moana Press 1986

### Jim Horton and Susan Jessie
**The Five Rhythms,** Gabrielle Roth **www.gabrielleroth.com**

## *Culture-making: What will a globally responsible world-view look like?*

**One Taste**, The Journals of Ken Wilber, Shambhala Publications 1999

## *Photographs*

Rose Diamond, page 23, 47, 137, 155, 267, 287
Siena Ammon, page 28, 312, 342
Henrique Araujo, page 51, 62, 85, 92, 94, 103, 113, 122/3, 167, 185,
    196/7, 242/3, 251, 293  www.henriquearuajo.com
Project Port Lyttelton,  page 143, 215, 231, 232, 235, 236
Photos of Earthsong by Robin Allison, page 221, 223, 226
Photo of Rose Diamond by Rosalyn Broas
Photo of Vivienne Wright by Jo Wickham Photography, Auckland
Photos of Hope by Daring Donna
Kids photos from Stephen Gordon, Sunnybrae Normal School, Auckland
Kids quotes: from Mary McQuoid and the children of Sherwood Primary
    School, Auckland

# TRANSFORMATIONAL TOOL BOX

*1. Resources*

*2. The Premises*

*3. Transformational Shifts*

*4. The Authentic Human*

*5. Values*

*6. The Pillars*

*7. Culture Making*

## *1. Resources*

These are just a few personal favourites, classics and recommended books, dvds and organisations arranged according to the six pillars of transformational learning.

**A. LIVING IN SERVICE TO HUMANITY, PLANET EARTH AND ALL LIVING SYSTEMS; HONOURING THE INTERCONNECTEDNESS AND SACREDNESS OF ALL LIFE**

**Books:**

**The Spell of the Sensuous, Perception and Language in a more-than-human World,** David Abram, Vintage 1996

**Celebrating the Southern Seasons, Rituals for Aotearoa,** Juliet Batten, Random House, NZ

**The Dream of the Earth,** Thomas Berry, Sierra Club Books 1998

**Other Ways of Knowing,** John Broomfield, Inner Traditions

**The Web of Life, A New Scientific Understanding of Living Systems,** Fritjof Capra, Doubleday 1996 **The Tao of Physics,** Fritjof Capra, Shambhala 1975

**Silent Spring,** Rachel Carson, Houghton Mifflin 1962

**The Cousteau Almanac, An Inventory of Life on our Water Planet,** Jacques Yves Cousteau 1980

**Deep Ecology, Living as if Nature Mattered,** Bill Devall and George Sessions, Gibbs M Smith 1985

**Pilgrim at Tinker Creek,** Annie Dillard, Harpers Magazine Press 1974

**Voluntary Simplicity,** Duane Elgin, Qill/Morrow 1993

**Natural Grace**, Matthew Fox and Rupert Sheldrake 1996

**The A.W.E. Project: Re-Inventing Education,** Matthew Fox 2006

**Toward a Transpersonal Ecology, Developing New Foundations for Environmentalism,** Warwick Fox, Shambhala 1990

**Woman and Nature: The Roaring Inside Her,** Susan Griffin, Harper and Row 1980

**The Last Hours of Ancient Sunlight, Waking up to Personal and Global Transformation,** Thom Hartmann, Mythical Books 1998

**The Ecology of Commerce**, Paul Hawken, HarperBusiness 1993.

**The Biophilia Hypothesis,** edited by Stephen R. Kellert and Edward O. Wilson, Island Press 1993

**Coming Back to Life: Practices to Reconnect our Lives, Our World,** Joanna Macy, New Society Publishers 1998

**World as Lover, World as Self,** Joanna Macy, Parallax 1991

**The End of Nature**, Bill McKibben, Random House 1989

**The Field, The Quest for the Secret Force of the Universe,** Lynne McTaggart, Harper Collins 2001.

**Permaculture: A Practical Guide for a Sustainable Future,** Bill Mollison, Island Press 1990. www.permacultureactivist.net.

**Inside the Animal Mind, A Groundbreaking Explanation of Animal Intelligence,** George Page, Doubleday 1999

**Where the Wasteland Ends (1973) PersonPlanet (1978) The Voice of the Earth (1992)** Theodore Roszak, Simon and Schuster

**Gaia: The Human Journey from Chaos to Cosmos:** Elisabet Sahtouris, Simon and Schuster 1989

**Thinking Like a Mountain: Toward a Council of all Beings,** John Seed, Joanna Macy, P. Fleming and A. Naess, New Society Publishers 1988

**The Rebirth of Nature, The Greening of Science and God**, Rupert Sheldrake, Century 1990

**The Fifth Sacred Thing,** Starhawk, Bantam 1993 and **Walking to Mercury,** Bantam 1997 (novels).

**A New Earth: Awakening to your Life's Purpose,** Eckhart Tolle, Dutton/ Penguin 2005

**Secrets of the Soil, New Age Solutions for Restoring our Planet,** Peter Tompkins and Christopher Bird

**The Journals of Henry D. Thoreau 1837-1852**, Princeton University Press

www.wiserearth.org - a networking website run by the Natural Capital Institute.

**Dvds: The Gathering: Return of the Whale Dreamers** www.whale-dreamers.com

**Who's Counting: Marilyn Waring on Sex, Lies, and Global Economics**, Terre Nash, National Film Board of Canada, 1995. A powerful film about New Zealand ex-Member of Parliament, Marilyn Waring and her investigation into how economic measurements discount the work of women and nature.

## B. INNER WORK

**Books:**

**The Inner Journey Home, Soul's Realization of the Unity of Reality,** A.H. Almaas, Shambhala 2004

**Facets of Unity**, A H Almaas, Diamond Books 1988

**Iron John, A Book about Men,** Robert Bly, Da Capo Press 2004

**The Power of Myth**, Joseph Campbell and Bill Moyers, Doubleday 1988

**When Things Fall Apart, Heart Advice for Difficult Times** 1994 , **No Time to Lose, A Timely Guide to the way of the Bodhisattva** 2005, **Practicing Peace in Times of War**, Pema Chodron, Snow Lion Publications

**Be Here Now,** Anchor Books 1969 and **Journey of Awakening: A Meditator's Guidebook,** Ram Dass, Bantam Books 1978

**Migration to the Heartland, a Soul Journey in Aotearoa,** Rose Diamond, Heart and Soul 2004

**Women who Run with the Wolves**, Clarissa Pinkola Estes, Ballantine 1992

**The Diamond in your Pocket**, Gangaji, Sounds True 2005

**Dynamics of the Unconscious**1988, **Development of the Personality** 1987, Liz Greene and Howards Sasportas, Weiser (astrology/mythology)

**Spiritual Emergency, When Personal Transformation becomes a Crisis**, Stanislav and Christina Grof, Tarcher/Putnam 1989 **The Stormy Search for the Self,** Stan Grof

**Being Peace,** Thich Nhat Hahn, Parallax Press 1987 and **Love in Action**

**The Way of the Shaman,** Michael Harner, www.shamanism.org

**The Eye of the I, From Which Nothing is Hidden,** David Hawkins, Veritas Publishing 2001

**After the Ecstasy, the Laundry**, Jack Kornfield, Bantam 2000

**Who Dies? An Exploration of Conscious Living and Conscious Dying,** Stephen Levine, Doubleday 1982

**The Intention Experiment, Using your thoughts to change your life and the world,** Lynne McTaggart, Free Press 2007

**Enlightenment, the Yoga Sutras of Patanjali**, MSI, SFA Publications 1995

**The Tibetan Book of Living and Dying,** Sogyal Rinpoche, Harper Collins 1992

**Love and the Soul, Creating a Future for Earth**, Robert Sardello, Harper 1995

**The Power of Now**, Eckhart Tolle, Hodder 1999

**Grace and Grit, Spirituality and Healing in the Life and Death of Treya Killam Wilber,** Ken Wilber, Shambhala 1991

**The Seat of the Soul**, Gary Zukav www.zukav.com

**CDs:**
**Waking from the Trance, A Practical Course for Developing Multi-Dimensional Awareness,** Stephen Wolinsky, Sounds True 2001
www.shambhala.com
www.soundstrue.com

## C. CONSCIOUS RELATIONSHIP
**The Way of the Superior Man**, David Deida, Sounds True 2004
**Fatherless Sons: The Experience of New Zealand Men,** Rex McCann, Harper Collins, www.essentiallymen.net
**The Virtues Project,** The Family Virtues Guide, Penguin 1997, Family Virtues Cards, Virtues Reflection Cards, **Linda Kavelin Popov, Dan Popov, John Kavelin** www.virtuesproject.com
**The Dream of a Common Language,** and **A Wild Patience Has Taken me this Far**, Adrienne Rich, Norton and Co. (poems)
**Speaking Peace,** Marshall Rosenberg, Sounds True, 2003, www.CNVC.org
**Non Violent Communication,** Marshall Rosenberg, PuddleDancer Press 2005
**The Four Agreements**, Don Miguel Ruiz, Amber-Allen, 1997 and **The Mastery of Love**
**The Power of Now,** Eckhart Tolle, Hodder 1999
**Turning to One Another: Simple Conversations to Restore Hope to the Future**, Margaret Wheatley, Berrett-Koehler 2002, www.turning-tooneanother.net.
**Perfect Love, Imperfect Relationship; Healing the Wound of the Heart; Journey of the Heart, Path of Conscious Love; Love and Awakening, Discovering the Sacred Path of Intimate Relationship,** John Welwood

## D. LIVING YOUR PASSION:
**Creativity:**
**The Four-Fold Way: Walking the Paths of the Warrior, Teacher, Healer and Visionary,** Angeles Arrien, 1993 www.angelesarrien.com
**On Creativity,** David Bohm, Routledge 2004
**The Artist's Way, A Spiritual Path to Higher Creativity,** Julia Cameron, Tarcher/Putnam 1992
**The Seven Spiritual Laws of Success,** Deepak Chopra, Bantam 1996
**Creativity** and **Flow,** Mihaly Csiksentmihalyi, Harper Collins 1996
**The Spirit of Creativity, Thoughts on Living One's CreativeTruth,** Joseph Curiale, Xlibris Corp 2006
**A Flash of Lightning in the Dark of Night, a Guide to the Bodhisattva's Way of Life,** The Dalai Lama, Shambhala Dragon 1994
**How Can I Help? Stories and Reflections on Service,** Ram Dass and Paul Gorman, Alfred A. Knopf 1987

**The Power of Intention,** Wayne Dyer 2005

**Making a Living While Making a Difference,** Melissa Everett. www.sustainablecareers.com

**Creativity: Where the Divine and the Human meet,** Matthew Fox, Tarcher/Putnam 2002 www.matthewfox.org

**Creating: A practical Guide to the Creative Process and How to use it to Create Anything,** Robert Fritz, Ballantine Books 1993; **Your Life as Art,** Robert Fritz, New Fane Books 2002 www.robertfritz.com

**Excuse Me Your Life is Waiting,** The Astonishing Power of Feelings, Lyn Grabhorn, Hampton Roads 2003

**The Tenth Insight: Holding the Vision, an Experiential Guide**, James Redfield and Carol Adrienne, Warner Books 1996

**Everyday Miracles: The Inner Art of Manifestation**, David Spangler, Bantam 1996.

**Creative Process in Gestalt Therapy,** Joseph Zinker, Vintage Books 1978


**Support for Social Entrepreneurship:**

**Changemakers 5-10-5-10 webinquiry@changemakers.org.nz**

Since 2006, several groups from around New Zealand have been developing a new style of community group which aims to inspire and support a greater citizen engagement on social, economic and environmental issues.

**The New Zealand Social Innovation Investment Group** and **The New Zealand Social Entrepreneur Fellowship** www.nzsef.org.nz

Brought together in 2006 by Stephen Tindall, founder of the Tindall Foundation, this is a key group of grant-makers, philanthropists and philanthropic representatives who are learning how to more effectively support social entrepreneurship in New Zealand. The Group seeks to connect leading New Zealand social entrepreneurs with one another; learn through the establishment of a social entrepreneur learning community; invest through directly matching social entrepreneurs with local philanthropy; develop the next generation of social entrepreneurship in New Zealand


**And globally:**

**Ashoka** strives to shape a global, entrepreneurial, competitive citizen sector; one that allows social entrepreneurs to thrive and enables the world's citizens to think and act as change makers. www.ashoka.org

**Social Edge:** a global blog full of interesting articles and some useful tips on how to write funding applications. www.socialedge.org

**Zaadz:** An inspirational online global community of leaders, visionaries, thinkers, artists, writers, healers, teachers, activists, environmentalists, conscious entrepreneurs and many others. Zaadz includes people of

many ages (from 12 to 90), many nationalities, from over 100 different
countries and different backgrounds, some are already making huge
differences in thousands of lives, while others are working to make a
difference starting with themselves. www.zaadz.com

**The XL Results Foundation:** a global network for conscious entrepreneurs
and social enterprise. www.xresultsfoundation.com

There are also numerous community and trust funds available.

## E. CO-CREATIVE COMMUNITY

**Working Together, Producing Synergy by Honouring Diversity**, Angeles
Arrien (ed)

**The Tao of Democracy, Using Co-intelligence to Create a World that
Works for all,** Tom Atlee, The Writers' Collective 2003
www.taoofdemocracy.com www.co-intelligence.org

**Calling the Circle: The First and Future Culture,** Christina Baldwin,
Bantam 1998.

**Strong Democracy: Participatory Politics for a New Age,** Benjamin
Barber, University of California 1985

**On Dialogue,** David Bohm , Routledge 1996 www.david-bohm.org

**The World Café: Shaping our Future through Conversations that
Matter,** Juanita Brown, David Isaacs, Margaret Wheatley, Peter Senge.

**Appreciative Inquiry: The Handbook** , David Cooperrider and Diana
Whitney, Lake-shore 2001. www.appreciativeinquiry.cwru.edu.

**The Chalice and the Blade**, Riane Eisler, Harper and Row 1987. **The
Partnership Way: New Tools for Living and Learning, Healing Our
Families, Our Communities and Our World** HarperSanFrancisco 1990

**The Aquarian Conspiracy: Personal and Social Transformation in the
1980s**, Marilyn Ferguson Tarcher 1980.

**Pedagogy of the Oppressed,** Paulo Friere, Penguin 1972.

**Blessed Unrest, How the Largest Movement in the World Came into
Being and Why No One Saw it Coming.** Paul Hawken, Viking Press
2007

**Building a Win-Win World: Life Beyond Global Economic Warfare,**
Hazel Henderson, Berrett-Koehler 1996.

**The Change Handbook: Group Methods for Shaping the Future,** Peggy
Holman and Tom Devane (eds) Berrett-Koehler 1999.

**The Politics of Meaning: Restoring Hope and Possibility in an
Age of Cynicism,** Michael Lerner, Addison-Wesley 1996. **Spirit
Matters,**Walsch Books/Hampton Roads 2000.

**Dialogue: Rediscovering the Transforming Power of Conversation,** Linda
Ellinor and Glenda Gerard, J. Wiley and Sons 1998.

**Co-operative Inquiry, Research into the Human Condition,** John Heron,
www.human-inquiry.com

**Dialogue, the Art of Thinking Together,** Wiliam Isaacs

**Grounding Vision—Empowering Culture: How to build & sustain community together. A Manual of Participatory Tools for Social Change Facilitators,** Robina McCurdy, Earthcare Education Aotearoa

**Spiritual Politics: Changing the World from the Inside Out,** Corinne McLaughlin and Gordon Davidson Ballantine Books, 1994.

**The Deep Democracy of Open Forums: Practical Steps to Conflict Prevention and Resolution for the Family, Workplace and World,** Arnold Mindell, Hampton Roads 2002. **Sitting in the Fire: Large Group Transformation Through Diversity and Conflict** Lao Tse Press 1997.**The Leader as Martial Artist,** HarperSF 1992.

**Open Space Technology: A User's Manual,** Harrison Owen, Berrett-Koehler 1997. See also www.openspaceworld.org.

**By Life's Grace: Musings on the Essence of Social Change,** Fran Peavey, New Society 1994; **Heart Politics,** New Society 1986.

**The Cultural Creatives: How 50 Million People are Changing the World,** Paul H Ray and Sherry Ruth Anderson, Harmony 2000. www.culturalcreatives.org.

**Presence: Human Purpose and the Field of the Future,** Peter Senge, Otto Scharmer Joseph Jaworksi, Betty Sue Flowers

**Synchronicity, the Inner Path of Leadership,** Jaworksi, Flowers and Senge

**The Fifth Discipline: The Art and Practice of the Learning Organization,** Peter Senge Doubleday Currency 1990. **The Fifth Discipline Fieldbook,** Doubleday Currency 1994.

**Creating Community Anywhere: Finding Support and Connection in a Fragmented World,** Carolyn Shaffer and Kristin Anundsen, Tarcher/Perigree 1993

**The Different Drum, Community Making and Peace,** M Scott Peck, Simon & Schuster 1987. **Going Local: Creating Self-Reliant Communities in a Global Age,** Michael Shuman, The Free Press 1998

**Truth or Dare: Encounters with Power, Authority and Mystery,** Starhawk, Harper and Row 1987.

**A Time for Choices: Deep Dialogues for Deep Democracy,** Michael Toms, New Society 2002.

**Turning the Century: Personal and Organizational Strategies for Your Changed World,** Robert Theobald, Participation 1992. **Reworking Success,** New Society 1997. www.resilientcommunities.org.

**Finding our Way, Leadership for an Uncertain Time** and **A Simpler Way,** Margaret Wheatley**Future Search: An Action Guide to Finding Common Ground in Organizations and Communities** , Marvin Weisborn and Sandra Janoff, Berrett-Koehler 1995. www.futuresearch.net.

**Community Financing:**

**Catherine Austin Fitts,** Navigating toward a more financially intimate world. www.solari.com

**Living Economies Aotearoa/New Zealand** www.le.org.nz includes a great resource section.

**The GreenMoney Journal,** www.greenmoney.com encourages and promotes the awareness of socially & environmentally responsible business, investing and consumer resources.

**The Soul of Money,** Lynne Twist www.soulofmoney.org

## 6. A SHARED STORY OF OUR ORIGINS, A CREATION CENTRED SPIRITUALITY

**Song of the Old Tides** and **Song of the Stone,** Barry Braislford www.stoneprint.co.nz **The Making of Tomorrow,** DVD

**Thank God For Evolution! How the Marriage of Science and Religion Will Transform your Life and our World,** Michael Dowd, Council Oak Books 2007

**Awakening Earth: Exploring the Evolution of Human Culture and Consciousnes,** Duane Elgin, William Morrow 1993. **Promise Ahead: A Vision of Hope and Action for Humanity's Future,** HarperCollins 2000. www.awakeningearth.org

**Original Blessing: a Primer in Creation Spirituality,** Matthew Fox, Bear and Co. 1983

**Conscious Evolution: Awakening the Power of Our Social Potential,** Barbara Marx Hubbard, New World Library 1998. **Humanity Ascending,** a dvd series, www.barbaramarxhubbard.com

**God and the Evolving Universe,** James Redfield, Michael Murphy, Sylvia Timbers, Tarcher/Putnam 2002

**Brief History of Everything,** Ken Wilber, Shambhala 1996, **Sex, Ecology, Spirituality: The Spirit of Evolution,** Shambhala Publications 1995, **Up from Eden, A Transpersonal View of Human Evolution,** Shambala 198,1 Ken Wilber, www.kenwilber.com

**Organisations promoting conscious evolution:**
www.andrewcohen.org/blog: Andrew Cohen
www.integralworld.net : Ken Wilber
www.wie.org: What is Enlightenment?
www.noetic.org: Institute of Noetic Science
www.co-intelligence.org: Co-Intelligence Institute
www.context.org: Context Institute
www.bethechange.org.uk: Be the Change/Change the Dream
www.evolve.org: Foundation for Conscious Evolution
www.oasishumanrelations.org.uk: Oasis School of Human Relations
www.findhorn.org: The Findhorn Foundation
www.schumachercollege.org.uk : Schumacher College
www.ridhwan.org: The Ridhwan Foundation (The Diamond Approach)
www.heartpolitics.net : Heart Politics
www.onenessuniversity.org : Deeksha/Oneness Blessing
www.artofliving.org: Art of Living Foundation

## *2. The Premises*

**Some of the premises upon which this book is based:**

Consciousness shifts are central to transformation.

We are transitioning through profound global change.

We are being called to become One Global Family.

We each make a difference.

We can change our minds.

Consciousness is the transformational catalyst.

There is an evolutionary intelligence moving through us.

Becoming more conscious is a commitment to deepening self discovery.

We are spiritual beings and spirit is unlimited.

When we link heart to heart and mind to mind, we create One World.

We are part of a global movement.

Living our passion as Love-in-action is a way of service and compassion.

# 3. Transformational Shifts to the NEW CULTURE

The process of becoming Love-in-action, authentic and creatively empowered, is a journey of experiential learning leading to greater trust and awareness, and enabling the development of the skills, wisdom and compassion necessary to be of service. It involves many shifts of consciousness. Here are some of them:

**The shift from seeking satisfaction outside ourselves to an exploration of inner being and inter-being through a process of experiential learning.** Courageously following the call of the heart to discover one's authentic being is a healing journey into the unknown depths of self. Experiential learning is the process of expanding awareness, self knowledge and self responsibility through action, reflection, experimentation, honest communication and feedback. Rather than being solely focused on achieving goals and outcomes in the outer world, the process of learning becomes a primary source of meaning in life and the journey itself becomes the goal.

**The shift from the head to the heart; from fear to love; and ultimately to whole mind.** The journey from the head to the heart involves remembering who we truly are. At certain times in life, the heart feels the tug of the soul and hears the call to authenticity. When we choose to accept and respond to this call, we begin the journey to greater awareness and heightened consciousness. We achieve our ultimate power and creativity when heart and mind are in balance, working together in harmony, and able to synthesize diverse elements into more inclusive wholes.

**The shift from feeling trapped by circumstances, to the recognition life is a journey of courage trust and discovery, and we are creators capable of making conscious choices.** When we hear the call of the inner life, and set out on our journey to find life's meaning and purpose, we learn to travel in deeper and more radical trust, shedding old psychological skins and our need to be in control. As we become simpler, we experience at a deeper level, our essential loving nature and the interconnectedness of everything. We realize there are myriad possibilities latent in each moment, and peace of mind and fulfillment rest, not so much in having what we want, as in consciously choosing to be aligned with authentic values.

**The shift in choosing to withdraw our energy from what is not working and instead put our attention on what we choose to create.** Focusing primarily on what is not working in the world, or in our personal lives, leads to cycles of reactivity and disempowerment. When we choose to use our dissatisfactions to fuel our passion for positive change, and focus wholeheartedly on what we choose to create, in alignment with higher values, we become pro-active and maximally empowered.

**The shift from relying on outer authorities, to connecting instead with inner guidance, authentic values and creativity.** As we commit to self awareness, self knowledge and self responsibility we learn to be present, to listen inwardly and trust our intuition. As if by magic, everything we need for the next step of our learning "shows up", even though we may not always recognize, nor greet people or events with open arms. The synchronicities of life reveal an intrinsic harmony, which in turn may lead to a deepening trust in, and curiosity about, the unfolding creative process of life.

**The shift from an illusion of separation and a belief we have to "do it alone" to the realization we are participating in an intelligent, abundant and friendly universe, which is calling us to be of service to the whole.** Becoming more inwardly satisfied and consciously focused on creativity, we experience at a deeper level the interconnected web of consciousness that runs through all life. As we develop acceptance and love for our own nature, the profound abundant generosity of life is revealed.

**The shift from self interest and exploitation to the choice to live in harmony.** With the realization of the essential interconnectedness of all life comes a responsibility to be of service to our interconnection. Living our passion as Love-in-action, we choose to exercise our creative freedom most fully through taking responsibility. Thus we become participants and co-creators in a creative universe.

**The shift from identifying with our thoughts, to recognizing we are not our thoughts and committing to mastering our minds.** The realization there is intelligence beyond individual mind, more powerful than thought, awakens us to a new dimension of consciousness and the recognition we are not who we thought we were. We may then choose to develop a discipline which supports us to withdraw our attention from negative thinking and limiting belief patterns in order to focus attention on our creative powers.

**The shift from feeling separate, to deciding to build sustainable co-creative community, wherever we happen to be.** Recognizing the power of grassroots change, and the necessity for us all to learn to live together and get along, we begin to create community wherever we are. Opportunities arise for accelerated creativity and learning, mutual support, conscious relationship, and sharing resources. We accept the challenge to bring forth new attitudes, skills and creative solutions to humanity's problems.

**The shift from businesses which create huge profits for a few whilst destroying the environment, to new sustainable models of business which honour life and give back to communities.** The creative impulse to discover and invent new solutions to shared problems frequently involves freeing energy which has become stuck in established forms and opening to more inclusivity. Social entrepreneurs are developing new business models based on the principles of natural abundance, unity in diversity and community service.

**The shift from concepts of "mine" and "yours", to recognition that the Universe is a constant flow of energy, and giving and receiving are one.** Learning to work with universal flow is possibly one of the most invigorating aspects of the emerging culture and certainly one of the most challenging for Westerners, particularly when it comes to sharing money and resources. As social entrepreneurs lay the tracks for the emergence of a new culture based on universal principles and values, growing numbers of philanthropists are recognizing their part in supporting such projects, and together they are building new alliances which strengthen the web of community.

**The shift to the realization of Unity.** We come to understand at a conceptual and intuitive level that every living being is connected into one indivisible and interdependent web of Life. Over time, and with meditative practice, this becomes an experiential, moment to moment realization of the Unity of all life. Or, a sudden peak experience may reveal this unity, and then we strive to integrate this new understanding with our established world view.

## 4. The Authentic Human

### *Living your Passion is a journey to becoming an authentic human being or being Love-in-action.*

Authentic human beings:

# Know who they are

Value life in all its manifestations

Know all life is essentially one interconnected whole

Give priority to self actualisation and higher consciousness

Listen to and follow inner guidance/ intuition rather than external rules and expectations

# Are self responsible

Understand life to be a process of experiential learning leading to greater wisdom and harmony

Are committed to keeping their own consciousness and energy in balance and well being

Realize that change on the outside starts with change on the inside

Take responsibility for their thoughts, emotions, and deeds

# Are creative

Value creating, sharing and service over accumulation

Are willing to take risks and live with uncertainty

Develop an attitude of detachment from outcomes

Love to live on their growing edge and expand their consciousness

Realize that all creation is co-creation

## 5. *Some Qualities and States of the Evolutionary Consciousness*

LOVE
PRESENCE
AWARENESS
TRUTH
TRUST
VIBRANCY
SPACIOUSNESS
CREATIVE FREEDOM
EMPOWERMENT
SURRENDER
TRANSFORMATION
WHOLENESS
EXPLORATION, ADVENTURE, DISCOVERY
JOY
RYHTHM
EQUILIBRIUM
CONSCIOUS PARTNERSHIP
EQUALITY
EXPERIENTIAL LEARNING
DIFFICULTIES ARE OPPORTUNITIES
COMPASSIONATE COMMUNICATION
SERVICE
HARMONY WITH NATURE
SIMPLIFICATION
STILLNESS
OBSERVATION
LISTENING
NON- ATTACHMENT
UNITY

## *6. THE PILLARS*

*A Shared Story Of Our Origins And The Evolution Of The New Universal Human, A Creation Centred Spirituality*

INNER WORK

CONSCIOUS RELATIONSHIP

LIVING YOUR PASSION

CO-CREATIVE COMMUNITY

**Living In Service To Humanity,
Planet Earth And All Living Systems**

**Honouring The Interconnectedness
And Sacredness Of All Life**

**Evolving Through Experiential Learning**

# 7. Culture-Making:
## The New Globally Responsible Culture
### Some constructive skills and attitudes

**We develop authentic power and creativity through:**

A daily consciousness practice

Controlling the mind

Aligning with higher values

Witnessing and surrender

Joy and gratitude

Going with the flow

A Whole New Worldview


**We develop conscious co-creative relationship through:**

Mirroring our divine nature to each other

Seeing difficulties as stepping stones

Practicing compassionate nonviolent communication

Participating in abundance

Synergistic co-creation with spirit


**We live gently on the Earth through:**

Natural methods of cultivation

Sustainable housing

Voluntary simplicity

Sharing resources

Waste minimisation


**As we heal the past we move on to build community in new ways by:**

Learning nonviolent communication skills

Encouraging inter-generational learning

Learning how to listen and find a common language

Valuing young people and training young leaders with heart

Negotiating for win-win solutions

Growing grassroots leadership

**Developing a healthier society and a global world view starts with respecting, valuing and celebrating difference by:**

Allowing people to meet their needs and create their own solutions in their own ways

Offering choices which reflect differences

Preserving diverse languages and ways of knowing

**Peace consciousness develops from our common human desire to be liked, understood and respected and is helped by:**

Coming together in harmony around common evolutionary goals

Nurturing global citizens

Creating forums for sharing dreams

Celebrating difference and sharing resources

Creating Rites of Passage to mark our transition to global consciousness.

**We mobilise for social justice through:**

Social networking on the web.

# *ACKNOWLEDGEMENTS*

I feel deeply privileged to have been able to write this book and very mindful of the rich resource of support that has held and fed me while I did so. Without the love, friendship, encouragement, willingness and work of many people, the book would not have come into being. My heartfelt gratitude goes to:

Maggie Holling; you were my mainstay and co-conspirator during 2006, while I did the work which seeded this book. Thank you so much for friendship, deep conversations, healing, financial support, and your wonderful cakes.

To Daring Donna and everyone at Swanson Sanctuary, where I conducted the first interviews, thank you for sanctuary and inspiration. Donna, Kristina Menheere and I sowed the seed for Rose Coloured Glasses, an adventure in co-creation through publishing, and Donna and Krissy held me with love and encouragement through the writing of the book whilst laying the groundwork for the New Zealand distribution.

My dear soul friend, Woods Elliott; thank you so much for your unfailingly enthusiastic encouragement for my writing and your unstinting devotion to reading, re-reading and editing; for the hours and hours of creative conversations; and most of all for providing me with a safe nest in Virginia USA, where I had nothing else to do but write. I am deeply grateful for your generosity and your willingness to see, support and participate in the vision.

To each one who gave the wonderfully inspiring interviews which kept me buoyed up, motivated and devoted to my task, you are: Kat Burns, David Dwyer, Will Lau, Frank Cook, Jonathan Evatt, Mirjam Busch and Rudolf Jarosewitsch, John Massey, Anahata and Orah Ishaya, Daring Donna, Robin Allison, Margaret Jefferies, James Samuel, Robina McCurdy, Daniel Batten, Leanne Holdsworth, Chris and Takawai Murphy, Jim Horton and Susan Jessie, Vivienne Anne Wright.